HEALTH PSYCHOLOGY RESEARCH FOCUS

RELIGION AND HEALTH

THE PERSPECTIVE OF HAPPY SCIENCE MEDICINE

HEALTH PSYCHOLOGY RESEARCH FOCUS

Additional books in this series can be found on Nova's website under the Series tab.

Additional e-books in this series can be found on Nova's website under the e-book tab.

HEALTH PSYCHOLOGY RESEARCH FOCUS

RELIGION AND HEALTH

THE PERSPECTIVE OF HAPPY SCIENCE MEDICINE

YOICHI CHIDA, MD, PHD

NOVINKA

New York

NOTICE TO THE READER

Library of Congress Cataloging-in-Publication Data

Chida, Yoichi, 1972-
Religion and health : the perspective of Happy Science medicine / editors Yoichi Chida.
pages cm. -- (Health psychology research focus)
Includes bibliographical references and index.
ISBN 978-1-63483-401-8 (softcover)
1. Medicine--Religious aspects. 2. Spiritual healing. 3. Happy Science (Organization) I. Title.
BL65.M4C49 2015
299--dc23
2015026404

ISBN: 978-1-63483-401-8

Published by Nova Science Publishers, Inc. † New York

CONTENTS

List of Columns **ix**

Preface **xi**

Chapter 1 **Happy Science Doctrine** **1**

1. What Is Happy Science? 1

2. How Does Happy Science Bring Happiness? 2

3. Master Ryuho Okawa and the Supreme Being, El Cantare 3

3.1. Case Report 1 (Overcoming Father's Death) 5

4. Spiritual Views of Life 6

5. The Purpose of Living in this World 8

5.1. Case Report 2 (Near-Death Experience) 9

6. The Conscious and Unconscious 10

7. The Multidimensional Universe 10

7.1. Fourth Dimension 11

7.2. Fifth Dimension 11

7.3. Sixth Dimension 11

7.4. Seventh Dimension 12

7.5. Eighth Dimension 12

7.6. Ninth Dimension and Above 12

8. Guardian Spirits and Guiding Spirits 13

9. A Multi-Structured Spiritual Being 14

10. The Organs of Spiritual Bodies 15

10.1 Case Report 3 (Physical Reading) 16

11. The Mind Is the Main Controller 17

	References	17
Chapter 2	**Pathophysiology in Happy Science Medicine**	**21**
	1. The Relationship between Religion and Medicine	21
	2. The Key Role of the Mind in Diseases	22
	3. Happy Science's Views on Life and Death	23
	4. Physical Factors	24
	4.1. Lack of Exercise	24
	4.2. Poor Nutrition	25
	4.3. Physical Fatigue	25
	4.4. Poor Sleep Quality	26
	4.5. Genetic Factors	27
	5. Mental Factors	27
	5.1. Mental Function	27
	5.2. Mental States	28
	5.3. Malicious or Evil Spirit Possession	32
	5.4. Karma	39
	5.5. Case Report 4 (Soulmate)	40
	5.6. Teachers for Human Beings	44
	References	46
Chapter 3	**Medical Care in Happy Science Medicine**	**51**
	1. Medical Care Is Love	51
	2. Stages of Love	52
	3. Eightfold Path and Love	53
	4. Fundamental Love	56
	4.1. Having Spiritual Views of Life	56
	4.2. Smiling	57
	4.3. Gratitude	57
	4.4. Case Report 5 (Gratitude)	58
	5. Spiritually Nurturing Love	60
	5.1. Healthy Lifestyle	61
	5.2. Developing Problem-Solving Skills	61
	5.3. Strategic Withdrawals or Optimalism	62
	5.4. Case Report 6 (Perfectionism)	63
	6. Forgiving Love	65
	6.1. Detaching from Greed	65
	6.2. Forgiveness	66
	6.3. Developing Altruism	67

7. Love Incarnate 68
7.1. Positive Willpower 68
7.2. Faith and Prayer 69
7.3. Case Report 7 (Faith and Prayer) 70
7.4. Meditation 72
7.5. Collapse of Karma 73
References 74

Index **79**

LIST OF COLUMNS

Column 1	Stroke and Coronary Heart Disease	**29**
Column 2	Breast Cancer, Uterine Cancer, and Uterine Myoma	**30**
Column 3	Atopic Dermatitis 1	**31**
Column 4	Presbyopia and Ureteral Stones	**31**
Column 5	Dementia	**32**
Column 6	Cancer 1	**36**
Column 7	Rheumatism	**36**
Column 8	Common Cold and Influenza	**37**
Column 9	Multiple Personality Disorder and Schizophrenia	**37**
Column 10	Cancer 2	**42**
Column 11	Birthmarks and Birth Defects	**42**
Column 12	Atopic Dermatitis 2, Asthma, or Bronchitis	**42**
Column 13	Phobia	**43**
Column 14	Gender Identity Disorder	**43**
Column 15	Abortion	**44**
Column 16	Autism, Asperger's Syndrome, and ADHD	**45**

PREFACE

Historically, religion and medicine have been strongly connected. In the West, Christian religious organizations built the first public hospitals, as early as the fourth century, and religious orders trained and registered doctors right up to the time of the Reformation. However, beginning in the seventeenth century, around the Enlightenment, there was a near complete separation between religion and medicine, as evidenced by the widespread cultural transition to using science and technology to explain disease and methods of healing. From this time onwards, there was a major focus on the physical management of disease, which left the spiritual and psychological approaches to be considered at best as alternative or complementary forms of medicine. Nonetheless, in more recent decades, views on this separation have swung back: various academics have begun exploring health care in Christianity and the other major world religions such as Buddhism and Islam.

This trend can be viewed as part of a larger movement to investigate the effects of religion on health in the field of complementary and alternative medicine (CAM). Such research is ongoing, but, to date, the mechanisms underlying the association between religion and health remain unclear[1]. For instance, the results of my meta-analysis[2] showed that religiosity/spirituality was longitudinally associated with reduced mortality in healthy population studies (combined hazard ratio = 0.82, 95% CI = 0.76–0.87, $p < 0.001$). However, in a subgroup analyses investigating the possible mechanisms, the protective effect of religiosity/spirituality in the initially healthy population

[1] For instance: Koenig, H. (2012). *Handbook of Religion and Health 2nd edition*. New York, NY: Oxford University Press.

[2] Chida, Y., Steptoe, A., Powell, L.H. (2009). Religiosity/Spirituality and Mortality: A Systematic Quantitative Review. *Psychotherapy & Psychosomatics*, 78, 81-90.

studies was independent of behavioral pathways (less smoking, less drinking, more exercising, and higher socioeconomic status), the emotional pathway of decreasing negative affect, and the social support pathway. A major reason for the lack of finding any mechanisms may be that the religion and health literature provides no unified theoretical or theological basis from which to identify such mechanisms. Thus, to address this gap, Chapter 1 of this book would like to briefly introduce the doctrine of Happy Science, a religious movement founded by Master Ryuho Okawa in 1986 that has since grown into one of the most influential religious organizations in Japan, with a member base from more than 100 countries worldwide. As you will see in Chapter 1, Happy Science theory has embraced the basic teachings of the major religions (e.g., Christianity, Buddhism, Islam, and Judaism) because Master Okawa is the core consciousness of El Cantare (the supreme God of the Earth), which is the same existence that many religions refer to as God. Moreover, this theory provides concrete tenets on the spiritual views of life, the purpose of living in this world, the structure of our mind and soul, and the relationships between mind and body.

As you will see in Chapter 2, the Happy Science theory on diseases suggests that 70% or 80% of diseases are caused almost exclusively by the state of mind. Master Okawa has detailed how almost all modern diseases are caused by three factors—what we eat, lack of exercise, and stress—which indicates that psychological factors have a much stronger impact on the etiology and prognosis of illness than any physical, environmental or genetic factors per se. One illness-causing psychological factor is our subconscious mind, which allows us to seek refuge in sickness. Another psychological factor is the three worldly delusions advocated by Buddhism: greed, anger, and ignorance. In the case of incurable diseases such as autoimmune diseases or amyotrophic lateral sclerosis, there are three main causes that carry spiritual significance: (1) possession by malicious or evil spirits, (2) karma engraved onto the soul before its birth on Earth, and (3) a physical disability arising from the soul's decision to inspire in others feelings of courage, joy, and a sense of life's purpose. The first and third factors have long been recognized by both Christianity and Islam, and the second one addressed in Buddhism and Hinduism. This chapter also provides some brief columns on Happy Science theory's explanations for diseases such as cancer, heart disease, dementia, infection, autoimmune disease in order to make this theory more understandable.

Chapter 3 explains the treatment theories and methods based on the basic tenets of Happy Science. In particular, since the Happy Science doctrine regards medical care as love, these treatment theories and methods are systematically introduced according to the stages of love: fundamental love (having spiritual views on life, smiling, and showing gratitude), spiritually nurturing love (having a healthy lifestyle, developing problem-solving skills, and making strategic withdrawals or adhering to Optimalism[3]), forgiving love (detaching from greed, forgiving, and developing altruism), and love incarnate (using positive willpower, faith and prayer, meditation, and collapse of karma). In addition, throughout this book, I have provided case reports that make it easier to imagine how those with severe disorders can be miraculously cured through Happy Science Medicine. Taken together, the Happy Science perspective can account for the complementary relationships that exist between modern medicine and religion. Happy Science Medicine could be thus defined as an exquisite merger of the Happy Science doctrine with modern medicine, making it inconsistent with the thus-far conventional flaws of religion and health.

Yoichi Chida, MD, PhD
Faculty of Human Happiness,
Happy Science University
Department of Medical Science,
Happy Smile Clinic
Faculty of Human Happiness Office 4,
Happy Science University 4F,
4427-1 Hitomatsuhei, Chosei-mura, Chosei-gun,
Chiba 299-4325, Japan
E-mail: yoichi.chida@gmail.com

[3] Optimalism is a philosophical form of optimism, which specifically refers to a belief that while the world may not be perfect it is better than the available alternatives. The Optimalist understands that failures in life are part of the learning process, and appreciates the journey towards success.

Chapter 1

HAPPY SCIENCE DOCTRINE

1. WHAT IS HAPPY SCIENCE?

Happy Science, originally established in Japan as Kofuku-no-Kagaku (literally "the Science of Human Happiness") in 1986, has grown into one of the most influential religious organizations in Japan, and now includes members from over 100 countries worldwide. Indeed, the Agency for Cultural Affairs of the Japanese government reported approximately 11 million Happy Science believers, making it number one in the ranking of people who have joined Japanese religious groups (Agency for Cultural Affairs, 2014). Happy Science aims to empower individuals to discover happiness for themselves and to spread it to their families, communities, countries, and the world. Its grand mission is to create a utopia—a world filled with love, peace, harmony, and prosperity. The founder and leader is Master Ryuho Okawa, who, as of January 2015, has presented more than 2,200 lectures and authored over 1,700 books. His books have been translated into many languages, including English, German, French, Spanish, Portuguese, Hindi, Chinese, Nepali, Korean, Russian, Lithuanian, and Bulgarian, to reach as wide an audience as possible. Many of his books have reached the bestseller list, with some even selling millions of copies. His lectures have covered a wide range of genres and topics including life views, family issues, healing, business management, science, politics, economics, history, world affairs, and truths about the Spirit World and the universe (Happy Science, 2015).

2. How Does Happy Science Bring Happiness?

According to the basic tenets of Happy Science, universal happiness without the happiness of each individual is not possible, nor is personal happiness independent of the well-being of the whole. Each of us must first look within and take responsibility for our own happiness or unhappiness, which is the result of our thoughts and actions. The core teachings are known as the "Principles of Happiness," and consist of the fourfold path of "Love," "Wisdom," "Self-reflection," and "Progress" (Okawa, 2009a). Practicing the four Principles of Happiness is called "the exploration of the right mind." Individuals can begin with any principle that is appealing to them or that they think they must work on the most. From there, they will experience an upward spiral of spiritual growth.

The principle of Love is as follows: when we give love, we discover that our thirst for love and happiness is eased. Love is also to believe in other people. If people were children of the Devil, we would not love each other; however, people are the children of God. As such, we have to suppress some of our less admirable desires and be kind to those around us, and try to live a life that is of benefit to others and society as a whole. The principle of Wisdom is as follows: wisdom refers to deep life-knowledge and includes knowledge of spiritual facts and the Universal Truth. Knowledge is power. It provides us with the means to solve our problems and relieve us from our worries. Furthermore, by knowing the Truth, we can transform our lives by turning our former problems into highly rewarding experiences. These experiences will in turn allow us to speak wisdom to guide others. The principle of Self-reflection is as follows: many of us think that once a mistake is made, it is set in reality forever and cannot be altered. In a material sense, this is true. However, what happens in the mind encompasses the past, present, and future. When we regret and truly repent our actions, not only can the mistake be undone, but also we will receive blessings for awakening to the Truth that far outweigh what we had before. Genuine self-reflection can offer far more than simple forgiveness and provide support, encouragement, power, and energy. Finally, the principle of Progress is as follows: there are many methods to win or succeed, whether in business or in life. The law of thought is that both good and bad thoughts will someday be manifested. By mastering love, wisdom, and self-reflection, we can put ourselves on the right path to progress, wherein the achievement of our goals contributes to the happiness of all humankind. Based on these principles, the members of my research group and I have already developed a novel religious/spiritual group psychotherapy and have reported its efficacy in treating various mental disorders in randomized controlled trials (Chida & Kim, 2011; Chida et al. forthcoming).

Happy Science believers receive a sutra book upon joining, "The Dharma of the Right Mind," and a set of prayer books. "The Dharma of the Right Mind" was inspired by Shakyamuni Buddha's consciousness and therefore has the power to purify minds with the light of Buddha. This prayer has been described as possessing 10,000 times more power than the Lotus Sutra or the Heart Sutra of Buddhism (Happy Science, 2015). Happy Science members' spiritual life, of which prayer constitutes a core component, revolves around the recitation of the sutras and prayers contained in these books.

3. Master Ryuho Okawa and the Supreme Being, El Cantare

Master Ryuho Okawa was born on July 7, 1956 in Tokushima Prefecture, Japan. On March 23, 1981, Master Okawa started communicating with the spirit world and attained Great Enlightenment. He awakened to the fact that he is the rebirth of Shakyamuni Buddha* and the core consciousness of El Cantare—the supreme God of the Earth.

Happy Science has a unique cosmology, proposing that the universe has a multi-dimensional structure. Within this structure, the material world is three dimensional, whereas the other world, the spirit world, refers to the fourth dimension and above. The spirit world of Earth spans up to the ninth dimension, which is the highest limit of personified spiritual existences. Happy Science believers believe in the existence of the Supreme Being, known as El Cantare, which is the same existence referred to in many religions (e.g., Christianity and Islam) as God. El Cantare is the leader of ten ninth-dimension spirits, including Jesus Christ, Confucius, Zeus, and Moses (Okawa, 2013). The name "El Cantare" means "the One," "the Beginning," "the Source," or "the Light of the Earth" (Okawa, 2011a). Indeed, Master Okawa has offered many teachings on this topic, including the following (pp.17-26 in Okawa, 2014a): "Today, Jesus is one of my best friends, but in a spiritual meaning, he

* The past incarnations of Ryuho Okawa's brother souls over the last 20,000 years include La Mu on the Mu continent, Thoth in Atlantis, Rient Arl Croud in the ancient kingdom of the Incas, Ophealis and Hermes in Greece, and Gautama Siddhartha (Shakyamuni Buddha) in India. The core consciousness of El Cantare has descended only three times in the 300 million years of the history of humanity, the third being Master Ryuho Okawa in the present day. The two previous descents were under the names Alpha and then Elohim.

is one of my famous disciples. This is very important and was a hidden secret in these thousands of years. And you came to know by Happy Science only, the real meaning of what he meant by 'Father.' His Father's name, his Father's spiritual name, was and is 'El Cantare.' That's a crucial point in my teachings. You should know that I am his Father. I guided him. I gave him many inspiration[s] and taught him the teachings of love. 'You should choose love.' That was my teaching at the time. Once, more than 3,000 years ago, I also said to Moses, 'I am that I am!' Do you know the meaning of 'I am that I am?' 'I am that I am' is 'I am the Being. I am the Origin. I am the origin of love.' That's the meaning of 'I am that I am.' [...]. In addition to that, around 600 A.D., there was Muhammad. Muhammad was a Muslim. In Islam, there is God, Allah. In the Koran, Allah said 'we.' Why did He say 'we''? In Islam He's the single God, but He said 'we.' 'We' means plural. There are many angels, guardian angels and guiding angels, in Heaven. More than 40 high-level angels were there and one of them taught Muhammad at that time. He knew him as Jibreel or Gabriel. One of the great angels. But these 40 angels were guided by El Cantare. I also sent Muhammad."

In another description of El Cantare, Master Okawa explained the following (Okawa, 2008a): "Then you might ask me, "Can you explain to me who the Lord is?" The being called Lord El Cantare, essentially, can never appear before people in visible form. Today, you have an extraordinarily rare chance in humankind's history to see El Cantare through me. However, under normal circumstances, El Cantare's existence is imperceptible outside the imagination. By this, I mean that in the other world, I no longer have arms, legs, and a face. I exist as light, nothing but light. In Buddhism, the Mahavairocana symbolizes Truth, and Amitabha is a representation of infinite light, compassion, and salvation. Lastly, the Shakya Tathagata represents Shakyamuni Buddha, the historical figure of Gautama Siddhartha. Although they are represented separately, they are all really the same. That is because the source from which they originate is divine light itself, which provides an infinite supply of light. In fact, it is the energy source supplying light to the spiritual sun, and it is the source of power that directs the terrestrial spirit group. El Cantare is the source of light; He is an existence without shape. Today, you have an opportunity to see a part of El Cantare in physical form but this is only for a brief moment within the course of human history. It is such a short moment, much like riding a speeding bullet train, and seeing from the window a glimpse of a poster on a utility pole. The chance which you have to see Him in real form is only for a quick, brief flash. Although my dharma lectures last about an hour, they last but a brief second in history. Please know that one lecture is a tiny little spark, an instant that flashes, and then, just as quickly, goes out. All of you must see the shadow of the eternal that is cast in this brief moment, take a hold of it, and keep it deep in your hearts."

3.1. Case Report 1 (Overcoming Father's Death)

In the following section, I describe the story of a Happy Science member (Saraphun Wongngernyuang, Thailand; Happy Science, 2014) in order to show how she encountered Happy Science's teachings and found happiness by overcoming her father's death.

When Saraphun was walking home after work, she passed by a branch of Happy Science, and the name 'Happy Science' caught her attention. At the time, she was longing for happiness and believed that there must be a practical way to achieve it. She picked up a brochure at the branch, which detailed the Principles of Happiness and the unity of religions. This answered the questions within her heart. "As a Catholic girl growing up in a Buddhist country, I couldn't help but doubt if the teachings of the two religions were compatible and if God would allow us to practice other religious practices. The answer I found in Master Okawa's teachings was simple—we are all from the same source, therefore, we should have respect for each other and try to understand the differences between religions. The more you study, the more you will find that all religions are compatible if you understand the teachings in the correct manner."

Saraphun felt she needed to search for something, so she left Thailand and moved to the United States to work as a server at her uncle's Thai restaurant. However, she was still unsure of what her true mission was and lost hope. That is when the name "Happy Science" popped up in her mind. She looked it up on the Internet, found their website, and bought Master Okawa's book, *Change Your Life, Change the World.* It changed her life. "After that I couldn't stop reading Happy Science books, one after another. I found the knowledge I needed to live life happily and overcome my struggles. I started to have hope again and believe that the future is going to be bright, starting with having a positive mindset." Things seemed to fall into place after that, but she still had difficulty finding her mission and knowing her true self. "What am I going to do in the future?" was always a big question on her mind; this is where meditation helped her.

"At the time, my father was suffering from liver cancer for which there was no cure. I realized that I needed to step up and become a leader with a positive attitude during the hard time when everyone in my family was miserable and thought that the sickness was a great misfortune. My father was already a Happy Science member, so I encouraged him to study about the relationship between the body and mind. One book that helped him a lot was *Healing Yourself*. He accepted that the sickness was not a misfortune, but an opportunity for him to refine his soul. I tried my best to guide him with Happy Science teachings on the meaning of life, the spirit world, and the aspiration for the future.

"He took the time when he was sick to reflect on himself, until he was able to let go of all his worries and found gratitude for the Lord for each day he was allowed to live. Also, [he expressed] gratitude towards family and friends, who had always given him support until the last day of his life. He told me that his wish was to help spread these great teachings and support the activities of Happy Science. Although his cancer was not cured, I am proud that he had a fighting spirit; he didn't give up and took his time to truly polish his mind. He left this world peacefully, knowing that he has completed his workbook of life.

"The Buddhist idea of 'the void' brought me a new perspective on life. As the important phrase goes 'matter is void, void is matter,' I came to realize that this world is only temporary, and what we can take with us after death is only our minds. Therefore, it's very important to pay attention to what is in our mind. Unless we have a mind of giving, we cannot truly say that we have led a fruitful life.

"I wish to do missionary work for Happy Science, spreading the truth all over the world, starting from my home country of Thailand. I have a dream to help light up the hearts and minds of those who are still living in delusion and help them lead a happy and prosperous life. I think it is important that we continue to 'Explore the Right Mind' every day and practice giving love to as many people as we can. I believe this will open doors to endless opportunities while we are living a beautiful life on Earth."

4. Spiritual Views of Life

In the Happy Science cosmology, human souls are repeatedly reincarnated for the purpose of spiritual evolution. The material world is considered a training ground for souls; as these souls evolve and begin to reach dimensions above the seventh, or the world of angels, they begin to act as guiding spirits.

In his book *"I'm Fine" Spirit: How to Get Through Tough Times*, Master Okawa talks about the spiritual views of life, as follows (page 56 in 2008b).

> "All human beings reincarnate in this world repeatedly to further their spiritual growth. If you try to see your spiritual training from this perspective, then what you originally saw as an ordeal will look different to you. You will realize that the problems you face right now reveal what kind of challenges you have to overcome in this life. Life is like a workbook of problems to be solved. So even if you feel that you are being swept away in a whirlpool of suffering, it actually means that you are facing one of the most important issues in your life, and you are currently experiencing a crucial time for your spiritual growth. This is an exciting time for you."

Reincarnation is ordinarily regarded as part of Eastern religious philosophy; however, there have been a number of scientific investigations on this topic in Western countries. For instance, more than 2,500 cases of children's memories of previous lives are registered in the files of the Division of Perceptual Studies at the University of Virginia. For more than forty years, the researchers have investigated these children's reports and concluded that they provide evidence that consciousness can survive death in at least some situations, which is surely a highly important finding. They also pointed out that this means that each of us is more than just a physical body (Tucker, 2005). Moreover, Past Life Therapy (PLT) has suggested the existence of reincarnation. PLT is a type of hypnotherapy devised by the psychiatrist Brian Weiss. The technique involves the client regressing, under hypnosis, back beyond birth (Weiss, 1996). It is said that in recollecting a past life, the client is healed by deepening his or her self-understanding and awareness of his or her current problems and can find the key to solving these problems. Notably, Christianity denies reincarnation, but Master Okawa has recorded a number of spiritual messages from Jesus Christ, such as the following (pp.16-20 in Okawa, 2014b): "I, myself, taught reincarnation about 2,000 years ago because I, myself, learned the religious teachings of Egypt. When I went on a trip and stayed in Egypt, I learned a lot about reincarnation from the priests of Egyptian temples. I also knew about reincarnation from the people who came to Egypt or Israel from India. There already were Buddhist temples in Egypt at that time and the disciples of Gautama Buddha came and taught about reincarnation. Also, we, the prophets of or before Christianity, accepted that 'the higher spirits or angels usually come down to Earth and save the people' was true. So, I, myself, taught you in the Bible that Elijah already came. I said, 'Elijah means John the Baptist. He's Elijah. He came already and I am the next one.' […]. Some people deleted the descriptions regarding reincarnations from the New Testament in the Bible, but I admitted it, of course."

5. The Purpose of Living in this World

The abovementioned investigations suggest that, after coming into being in this world, almost all of us forget knowledge of our previous lives and the spirit world. One could compare living in this world to living inside an aquarium—we are living in a place that is cut off from the true world.

Master Okawa has explained why this world was separated from the spirit world in the first place and why people are born into this world (pp.204-205 in Okawa, 2005): "If you look at it from the perspective of the spirit world, you will understand the reason. Actually, this world is a very good place to learn lessons for training the soul. The spirit world is a world of complete freedom, but if you are living there, it is hard to appreciate this spiritual freedom. It is only when you have been born on Earth that you can understand the value of this spiritual freedom. For that reason, despite all the pain it involves, you will choose to be reborn on Earth time and again. There are people who like running marathons, despite the rigor this involves, as well as people who like to swim, despite the exertion. They continue practicing because they wish to test their abilities within a given set of rules. Running twenty-six miles in a marathon, swimming, or practicing judo are all hard on the body, but people do not stop doing them. Why is this? It is because they wish to overcome handicaps and test the limits of their abilities. They wish to better themselves and win the respect of others. For the same reason, people are born into this world, this particular world. This system may appear strange, but the fact that our lifespan in this world is limited shows that God or Buddha has not set it up with an intention to punish us or make us suffer. It would be very mean of God or Buddha if we were sent to live on Earth forever when there is a world of freedom in the spirit world. But our time on Earth is limited. […]. Since you are only here for a limited time, you cannot understand all the truths of the world, and because you do not understand everything, you will make efforts to get to know them. As you live spiritually blind, you may go through numerous hardships, but it will give you a store of experience and strengthen your soul. It is similar to climbing a mountain; you choose to undergo difficulties and temper your soul."

5.1. Case Report 2 (Near-Death Experience)

In the following case, I relate how a Happy Science member (Emiko Hoshino, Japan; Happy Science, 2011) suffered a critical relapse of her illness and that, while in a coma for four long months, her soul travelled through the spiritual world.

By day, her father worked as a garbage collector for the city, but at night, he drank too much and became violent. They were very poor, and at school, other students often made fun of her, calling her, "the child of a garbage man." Her family's finances were a disaster, so she gave up going to high school and started working immediately after finishing middle school. She was married three times, but her husbands could not support her family and were even violent to her young daughters. Finally, she decided to raise these three children from different fathers on her own. When she was 29 years old, her sister invited her to visit the Yokohama temple of Happy Science. In October 1998, she became a believer of Happy Science. Since then, she has visited the temple almost daily and has consulted with the temple manager and staff members about her life. Furthermore, she learned Happy Science's truth.

It happened suddenly. In the spring of 2006, she was diagnosed with chronic myeloid leukemia. However, two to three days after receiving the prayer, "*Prayer for Recovery from Illness*," which her religious friends had recommended her, the doctor said that she was completely cured. From that point on, she was determined to live the rest of her life for others and enthusiastically took up missionary work. However, in 2009, the leukemia returned. Her religious friend always told her, "Ms. Hoshino, you need to rest," but she ignored her friend's advice and ended up suffering from overwork. In spite of receiving a bone-marrow transplant, her condition deteriorated and she soon became unable to speak clearly. She eventually fell into a coma.

While in a coma, she could see that many people were trying to crawl up out a large pit of quicksand. A lady called out to her, beseeching, "I did not do anything wrong! What is wrong about trying to get promoted? Isn't that something everyone wants?" Emiko guessed that the woman had fallen into that hell because she had lived her life only to get a promotion. In the next moment, countless photos began to continuously flow past Emiko, like a film. They were images depicting her entire life. When she stared at an individual photo, the time of her life from that photo began to play like a movie, beginning with that scene. She reflected on every single "picture" there and shed refreshing, revitalizing tears.

After about four months in a coma, she awakened. After further treatment and rehabilitation, in May 2010, she was finally able to leave the hospital. After over six months of battling the illness, she miraculously returned to her life.

6. The Conscious and Unconscious

Modern psychiatric medicine and clinical psychology use the concept of "the unconscious" and seek a scientific understanding of the mind via directing attention to its hidden depths and to the dynamic relations between the conscious and unconscious. It is largely associated with Sigmund Freud, but around the same time, Pierre Janet, Alfred Adler, and Carl Jung established their own forms of dynamic psychiatry. Some researchers have suggested that the Catholic exorcism marks the emergence of dynamic psychiatry (Ellenberger, 1970). Exorcism refers to a practice of ordering a demon to depart from a person in whom it was causing illness.

Considering the relationship between religion and health, the "universal unconscious" (or "collective unconscious"), as described by Jung in his investigations of the archetypes, is most germane here. This universality has sometimes been interpreted as the expression of a kind of neo-Platonic "world soul" or as the center of psychic energy (Ellenberger, 1970). In contrast, Master Okawa refers to "universal unconscious" as proof that all human beings are connected to each other, as well as with guardian and guiding spirits and even God, in what he calls a "great spiritual university" (Okawa, 2009b).

7. The Multidimensional Universe

The great spiritual university is suggested to be multidimensional (Okawa, 2013). In the context of the Happy Science theory, "dimensions" are ways of describing the characteristics of a specific world and its inhabitants according to how many traits they possess.

7.1. Fourth Dimension

In the fourth dimension (the Posthumous Realm), the element of time is added to length, width, and height. In our world, things that exist in the same general space will also exist in the same time, but this is not the case in the fourth dimension. It in the fourth dimension, two people shaking hands could be living in completely different periods in history. This dimension includes Hell, which is only a muddy lake that light does not reach. The negative energies within the atmosphere of Hell are envy; jealousy; reactive rage; excessive desire; dissatisfaction; pessimism; negativism; indecisiveness; cowardice; laziness; self-hatred; grudges; hatred; cursing; lust; aggression; egotism; abusive speech; deceit; manic depression; drunkenness; violence; exclusionism; lies; falsehood; materialism; atheism; alienation; authoritarianism; greed for money, status, and fame; and disharmony.

7.2. Fifth Dimension

The fifth dimension (the Realm of the Good) introduces the element of spiritual virtue. Its inhabitants are distinct not only in shape and the period to which they belong, but also in their level of spiritual awareness. Having some measure of spiritual awareness—that is, knowing that we are fundamentally spiritual beings—is a requirement for becoming an inhabitant of this world. This element of spirituality is principally measured by "goodness." Therefore, the fifth dimension is a world filled with virtuous people.

7.3. Sixth Dimension

Knowledge of the Truths is the additional element of the sixth dimension (the Light Realm), meaning that the inhabitants of this world differ in all the qualities of the fifth dimension, as well as in their knowledge of the Truths. The qualifications for living in the sixth dimension are virtue and having learned Buddha's teachings.

7.4. Seventh Dimension

In addition to differing in all the qualities of the sixth dimension, inhabitants of the seventh dimension (the Bodhisattvas Realm) differ in terms of the element of altruism. Inhabitants of dimensions below the seventh still live in a very self-focused way; this is not a judgment of them, but a simple observation. In the seventh dimension, their hearts are filled with love toward others, and all their deeds are selfless and in service of others. Inhabitants of this dimension are always giving love to each other and are actively instructing and guiding residents of lower dimensions.

7.5. Eighth Dimension

In the eighth dimension (the Tathagata Realm), compassion is added to the seven prior elements. Compassion is the desire to give unconditional mercy, and these higher sacred beings offer it freely, without reservation or distinction. While the love of the seventh dimension could be called the "love that gives," the love of the eighth dimension is even higher; it could be described as the "love that gives inexhaustibly." The love of the eighth dimension is never-ending, much like the sun; it is true compassion.

7.6. Ninth Dimension and Above

The ninth dimension (the Cosmic Realm) includes a new element called "cosmic universality." In the eighth dimension and below, inhabitants live within the multilayered structure of the planet Earth's spiritual field.

The ninth dimension, however, reaches beyond Earth's spiritual field, serving as the connection between our spirit world and those of other planets beyond our solar system. Thus, the inhabitants of this dimension guide Earth's spirit group based on an awareness of and involvement in spiritual evolution on a larger scale, as part of the greater cosmic universe. The deities of all world religions, who are considered the source of the Laws, inhabit this dimension.

Beyond the ninth dimension is the highest level of Earth's spirit group, the tenth dimension. None of the inhabitants of this realm are ever born as humans on Earth; in fact, they have no human character. There are only three spirits in the tenth dimension, who exist as separate consciousnesses. They take on primary roles in "creation" and "evolution." The three consciousnesses of the tenth dimension are the Sun Consciousness, Moon Consciousness, and Earth Consciousness.

Although the multidimensional world within Earth's system ends with the tenth dimension, there are other dimensions beyond it. The eleventh dimension is part of the multidimensional structure of the entire solar system, with a structural element called "the mission of the solar system." Beyond this is the galactic consciousness of the twelfth dimension, an unfathomably large spirit responsible for our galaxy. It is almost impossible to describe what lies beyond the twelfth dimension, but Master Okawa has said that the Primordial Buddha of the greater universe, the ultimate spiritual entity that we also call the Primordial God, most likely exists beyond the twentieth dimension.

8. Guardian Spirits and Guiding Spirits

Thanatological research by Kübler-Ross (1997) has suggested that every person has a guardian spirit or angel. These guardians assist us in the transition between life and death and help us choose our parents before we are born.

Master Okawa (2013) has explained about the system of guardian spirits and guiding spirits, who comprise spirits below the seventh dimension. As a general rule, these spirits form groups of six. The leader of each group is regarded as the "core spirit," and the other five are "branch spirits." All six spirits have the same tendencies and similar characteristics, and act in a manner similar to a human body, which also consists of six body parts: a head, two arms, a torso, and two legs. These six spirits take turns being born into this world to accomplish their life missions. Experience that any one spirit gains on Earth is shared with the other five spirits. In the past, the spirit who was next in line to be born acted as the guardian of the spirit ahead of it, who was already born on Earth. Nowadays, however, in order to cope with the complex structure of society, the spirit that was most recently incarnated takes the role of the guardian spirit so that it can provide guidance based on the most up-to-date information.

In addition, if a person on Earth has a critically important mission (e.g., governing a country or devising great products) to accomplish, he or she will be provided with a guiding spirit who specializes in that person's particular field.

9. A MULTI-STRUCTURED SPIRITUAL BEING

In Happy Science, a human being comprises more than just the flesh that we see with our eyes; each person is actually a multi-structured spiritual being that is temporarily residing in the physical body. The outermost layer of this spiritual structure is called the "astral body." The astral body actually has exactly the same shape and features as a human being (e.g., eyes, nose, eyebrows, heart, liver, and kidney) (Okawa, 2008c). Similar to this theory of a multi-structured spiritual being, early Egyptians believed that a person consisted of a physical body ("khat") and a soul. The soul consisted of three parts: the "ka," "ba," and "akh." The ka was believed to be an exact double of the person and was the life force that animated the body, which is quite similar to the function of the astral body. The ba was separate from the life force (ka), and survived after the body died. Given the right circumstances, however, the ka and ba would combine after death to form the akh. The akh "was the transfigured spirit that survived death and mingled with the gods." It was thought to survive in the afterlife only if the person had lived a good and worthy life (Wisseman, 2003).

Master Okawa provides a more detailed account of the theory of a multi-structured spiritual being, as follows (pp.163-165 in Okawa, 2005).

> "The details of our life in this world are recorded in what we call the 'astral body,' which envelops the 'spiritual body.' Souls remain inside this astral body for a certain period after death as they live in the Posthumous Realm of the fourth dimension. This astral body gives off vibrations that link the spirit world and Earth, so those in the fourth dimension generally live in this form. When souls move up from the fourth dimension to a higher realm, they slough off their astral body [...]. This astral body can be reused to create various phenomena in the Posthumous Realm* or reused by spirits from higher realms when they come down to visit Earth. It is also used as the basic material for the rebirth of a soul. [...]. Once the astral body has been cast off, there is the spiritual body, which exists beneath the astral body. It is a little more refined than the astral body. Souls live in this form in the fifth dimension and above. As souls move even higher and enter the realm of the Angels of Light, they find that even this spiritual body feels extremely heavy, like wearing a suit of armor, so it becomes necessary to remove yet another layer, to become an even more refined "light body," which is filled with a fair degree of light. They move on to live in the sixth dimension and beyond in

* Posthumous Realm means the fourth dimension

this light body. The worlds that exist beyond the sixth dimension have subtler vibrations and are more refined."

10. The Organs of Spiritual Bodies

Not only does every physical body contain an identically shaped spiritual body, every organ has its own corresponding spiritual version. In other words, the physical heart has a spiritual heart, the physical liver a spiritual liver, and the physical stomach a spiritual stomach, and so forth (Okawa, 2008c). Each of these spiritual organs has a different way of feeling because each has its own special mission and unique functions. For example, the spiritual stomach is extremely sensitive to emotions, and its sense of feeling is very acute. The spiritual heart feels on a much greater scale. In this manner, the spiritual organs are symbolic. When human beings experience considerable stress, the spiritual organs are the first to suffer damage (which organs are injured depends on the nature of the stress involved), after which the illness begins to manifest in the physical body as well.

Indeed, numerous clinical reports on organ transplants have shown how the physical and spiritual organs are related. Take, for example, the internationally famous case of Claire Sylvia in the USA (Sylvia & Novak, 1997): after a heart and lung transplant operation, she discovered that the new organs were not the only things she had inherited. While Claire had never liked foods such as beer and chicken nuggets, she suddenly started craving them after the transplant. Furthermore, several inexplicable changes in her personality occurred: she began looking at women in the way a man might, and her favorite colors became green and blue rather than the hot shades of pink, red, and gold she had once preferred. Months after the transplant, she had a dream about a young man called TL. When the dream was about to end, they kissed, and as their lips met, she seemed to inhale him, sucking his whole body into hers. She awoke convinced that a man named "Tim" was the donor of her heart and lungs. After this extraordinary dream, she sought out the family of her donor, who was a teenager named Tim Lamirande (initials TL) who had died in a motorcycle accident. She discovered that he had liked beer and had loved chicken nuggets; in fact, he had been carrying a box tucked inside his motorcycle jacket when he had crashed. His favorite colors were blue and green. This case suggests that it is possible for two souls to merge in one body, which indicates that every organ might have its own corresponding spiritual body part.

10.1 Case Report 3 (Physical Reading)

In public seminars on Happy Science, Master Okawa has conducted "physical readings," wherein he reads the feelings of a patient's organs using his spiritual abilities. This is much like what Edgar Cayce did—Cayce was an American mystic in the 20th century who allegedly possessed the ability to answer questions on various medical subjects by physical or karmic readings while in a trance (Karp, 1999). One of Okawa's sessions on a physical reading of a person's kidney is presented as follows (Okawa, 2011b).

"Questioner: I am in my 60s. Since I started running my own company at the age of 25, I have worked as a manager. At the time when I opened this business, I was hospitalized because of kidney disease for nine and a half months. Two years ago, a doctor declared, 'Your kidneys have begun to fail.' Nowadays, I think that, even while I fight against this disease, I want to complete my unfinished business. I would be really grateful if you could teach me the attitude necessary for me to accomplish this.

"Master Okawa: Yes, could you please keep standing up [from the speech table, Master Okawa holds both his hands up over the abdomen of the questioner, who is standing in the front row of the audience. He is silent for 5 seconds. Then, Master Okawa puts down his right hand and holds his left hand up]. Well. Right now, I am talking with your kidney. I am asking your kidney. It is saying, 'This person is working too hard.' Also, it is saying, 'Because he is overworking, my burden is very heavy.' Although you seem to work well, you have been straining yourself too much since starting your company. Because your working hours are too long, your burden of stress is heavy, and because you meet people so often, your intake of water such as tea is more than that of ordinary people, isn't it?

"Questioner: Yes. That's right.

"Master Okawa: It's twice that of ordinary people, isn't it?

"Questioner: Yes.

"Master Okawa: It might be, actually, more than twice that of ordinary people. You drink various things like green tea, coffee, and black tea, twice to three times as much as ordinary people. Since your kidney is working too much, it is tired. Your kidney is saying, 'I go beyond the usual capacity of the kidney to cope with water. Overintake of water is due to workplace stress and you depend on drinks for relaxation. So, you must sort out the stress.' I am compensating your kidney by proxy. Although your kidney also has a consciousness, it has no mouth. I feel very sorry for it, so I am compensating your kidney by proxy. Your kidney is saying, 'Since I understand well that you are trying to relax, you can drink something on occasion. But, could you please use a smaller cup? Your intake of water is too much. You may drink something many times, but please reduce the volume of the intake each time. Additionally, please increase the opportunities for sweating by exercising or physical labor.' This is what your kidney is saying."

11. The Mind Is the Main Controller

The mind, which has conscious and unconscious aspects, is the main controller of everything. Just as the physical heart acts as the core of the human body, the mind acts as the core of the soul (Okawa, 2013). The mind is not the brain or its cells, which is confirmed by the fact that even after we die and return to the spirit world, we retain every memory from our lives on Earth. The physical body that we leave behind eventually disappears from this world, but the soul and its core aspect, the mind, are always able to think, feel, and remember. A clear analogue is the relationship between a car and its driver, with the body being the car and the mind (or the soul) being the driver (Okawa, 2008d). The mind's thoughts influence the state of the astral body, which in turn determines the state of the physical body. When we allow negative thoughts such as anger, hatred, dissatisfaction, excess desire, pessimism, and a sense of inferiority to become concrete in our minds, these thoughts form a negative energy cloud. If those thoughts are only temporary, the negative energy will soon dissipate. However, when this energy persists for a certain length of time, it materializes and results in some form of illness. As such, those who suffer from illness have a part of their mind afflicted with negativity.

References

Agency for Cultural Affairs Japan. (2014). *An Almanac on Religion in 2014*. Available from: http://www.bunka.go.jp/shukyouhoujin/nenkan/pdf/h24 nenkan.pdf Accessed Feb 10, 2015 (Available only in Japanese).

Chida, Y., & Kim, Y. (2011). Chapter 10: Development of a Novel Spiritual Group Psychotherapy based on the Fourfold Paths: Happy Science Clinic Group Psychotherapy. In A.M. Columbus (Ed.) *Advances in Psychology*

Research Volume 81 (pp. 253-264). New York, NY: Nova Science Publishers Inc.

Chida, Y., Schrempft, S., & Steptoe, A. (In press). A novel religious/spiritual group psychotherapy reduces depressive symptoms in a randomized clinical trial. *Journal of Religion and Health.*

Ellenberger, H.F. (1970). *Discovery of the Unconscious.* New York, NY: Basic Books.

Happy Science (2011). Life Experience Stories. In Happy Science (Ed.) *The Spirit World Happy Science Monthly Issue 211.* Oct 2011.

Happy Science (2014). Member Story from Thailand. In Happy Science (Ed.) *Serenity Happy Science Monthly Issue 238.* Jun 2014.

Happy Science (2015). *Happy Science Official Homepage.* Available from: http://happy-science.org Accessed Feb 10, 2015.

Karp R.A. (1999). *Edgar Cayce Encyclopedia of Healing.* New York, NY: Grand Central Publishing.

Kübler-Ross, E. (1997). *The Wheel of Life: A Memoir of Living and Dying.* New York, NY: Scribner.

Okawa, R. (2005). *The Mystical Laws: Transcending the Dimensional Barrier.* Tokyo, Japan: IRH Press.

Okawa, R. (2008a). Chapter 2 Becoming Someone Who is Loved. In R. Okawa (Ed.) *My Lover, Cross the Valley of Tears* (pp. 53-77). Tokyo, Japan: Happy Science.

Okawa, R. (2008b). *"I'm Fine" Spirit: How to Get through Tough Times.* Tokyo, Japan: IRH Press.

Okawa, R. (2008c). Part III. The Power of Faith is the Key to Good Health. In R. Okawa (Ed.) *Healing Yourself: The True Relationship between Mind and Body* (pp. 187-225). Tokyo, Japan: IRH Press.

Okawa, R. (2008d). Part I. Building a Happy Relationship Between Mind and Body. In R. Okawa (Ed.) *Healing Yourself: The True Relationship between Mind and Body* (pp. 15-73). Tokyo, Japan: IRH Press.

Okawa, R. (2009a). Chapter 1 The Principle of Happiness. In R. Okawa (Ed.) *The Science of Happiness: 10 principles for manifesting your divine nature* (pp. 3-17). Rochester, VT: Destiny Books.

Okawa, R. (2009b). Chapter 4 The Way to Definite Health. In R. Okawa (Ed.) *The Way to Definite Health* (pp. 155-211). Tokyo, Japan: IRH Press. (Available only in Japanese and published with the Japanese title of "Chō Zettai Kenkō Hō" in 2009 by IRH Press).

Okawa, R. (2011a). *What is El Cantare-Belief?* Tokyo, Japan: Happy Science.

Okawa, R. (2011b). Chapter 4 Illness Reading (Q&A). In R. Okawa (Ed.) *The Miraculous Way to Overcoming Cancer* (pp. 135-175). Tokyo, Japan: IRH Press. (Available only in Japanese and published with the Japanese title of "Kiseki no Gan Kokufuku Hō" in 2011 by IRH Press).

Okawa, R. (2013). *The Laws of the Sun: One Source, One Planet, One People*. Tokyo, Japan: IRH Press.

Okawa, R. (2014a). *Be Positive*. Tokyo, Japan: IRH Press.

Okawa, R. (2014b). *Spiritual Messages From Jesus Christ*. Tokyo, Japan: Happy Science.

Sylvia, C. & Novak, W. (1997). *A Change of Heart*. New York, NY: Little, Brown & Company.

Tucker, J.B. (2005). *Life Before Life: A Scientific Investigation of Children's Memories of Previous Lives*. New York, NY: St. Martin's Press.

Weiss, B. (1996). *Many Lives, Many Masters: The True Story of a Prominent Psychiatrist, His Young Patient, and the Past Life Therapy That Changed Both Their Lives*. New York, NY: Grand Central Publishing.

Wisseman, S.U. (2003). *The Virtual Mummy*. Champaign, IL: University of Illinois Press.

Chapter 2

Pathophysiology in Happy Science Medicine

1. The Relationship between Religion and Medicine

The term "complementary" derives from the broader term CAM and refers to forms of treatment used in addition to standard or conventional therapies. This is distinct from alternative medicine per se, where conventional therapies are disregarded and replaced outright by alternative modalities. From the perspective of Happy Science, the relationship between religion and medicine is complementary. Indeed, Master Okawa has drawn attention to the complementary relationships that exist between modern medicine and religion, as follows (pp.222-225 in Okawa, 2008a):

> "How should we understand the relationship between modern medicine and religion? This is a challenging issue. I do believe that modern medicine is guided by the divine spirits. Here, let us call the angels of light in the field of medicine, 'Gods of Medicine.' When you trace the roots of the Gods of Medicine, you will eventually discover the god Hermes*. Eastern medicine sometimes conflicts with Western medicine, having originated in the classic

* Hermes: A god believed to have resided in Greece 4,300 years ago. Hermes is one of Master Okawa's brother souls and brought prosperity to the Mediterranean area, laying the foundations of Western civilization. He is well-known as the god of commerce, prosperity, the arts, travel, and communications, among others, Hermes is also the God of Healing. The Staff of Kerykeion (also known as the Caduceus), which Hermes is often depicted as holding, is used even today as a symbol of medical institutions worldwide.

> philosophies of Lao-tzu and Chuang-tzu, and Buddhism. There are actually many past examples in which monks taught medicine. The divine spirits are also providing ample guidance to religions that heal people's illnesses. From time to time, the divine spirits perform miracles to deepen people's faith. So, what is important is the cooperation and collaboration between medicine and religion. Physicians with religious faith should be able to heal more illnesses by effectively using the power of the mind. They should be able to miraculously cure even the most deadly illnesses by combining positive words and medicine. Likewise, people of religion should be capable of expanding the number of souls they save by cooperating with the positive side of medicine. The goal is people's happiness; therefore, cooperation is ideal."

Taken together, Happy Science Medicine could be defined as an ideal model combining modern medicine and religion, which treats disease both physically and spiritually by following the Happy Science doctrine described in Chapter 1.

2. The Key Role of the Mind in Diseases

From the perspective of Happy Science Medicine, 70–80% of diseases are caused almost exclusively by an individual's state of mind (Okawa, 2008b). It is important to realize that there is something within the individual that is causing the illness, which should be corrected first. Master Okawa has described this in more detail and has categorized diseases by their causal factors. Specifically, almost all modern diseases are caused by three factors: what we eat, lack of exercise, and stress (Okawa, 2008a). As mentioned before, the mind causes 70–80% of diseases; of these diseases, psychological stress and lifestyle behaviors cause 70–80% and 20–30%, respectively. Furthermore, Master Okawa has pointed out that even if individuals do not consciously believe that their failures or sins are forgiven by their suffering from sickness, this idea is present within their subconscious minds. People wish to fall ill, so they adopt unhealthy lifestyles and begin doing things that they should not do, pushing themselves to the limit until they collapse and fall ill (Okawa, 2008a). Thus, in a broad sense, even more than 80% of diseases might be caused by the state of mind.

Rare, incurable diseases such as leukemia and amyotrophic lateral sclerosis can be divided into the three categories by their cause (Okawa, 2008b): first are illnesses caused by karma engraved onto the soul before it was born on Earth. Namely, these patients have created the causes for their diseases in a previous life. Second are illnesses caused by evil spirits (i.e., possession). Finally are illnesses caused by individuals' own intention; that is, they have chosen their disability as part of their mission in order to inspire others with courage, joy, and a sense of purpose.

3. Happy Science's Views on Life and Death

Both medicine and religion deal with people existing on a borderline between life and death; thus, it is important to clarify Happy Science's views on life and death. Happy Science's views are actually quite similar to the story of the Cocoon & the Butterfly by Kübler-Ross (1997), in which death is simply a shedding of the physical body, much like the butterfly shedding its cocoon. Specifically, it is a transition to a higher state of consciousness where you continue to perceive, understand, laugh, and grow.

Master Okawa has explained the Happy Science's views on life and death in more detail, as follows (pp.65-68 in Okawa, 2008c): "The world beyond ours is in fact the real world, while this world is only temporary. This world exists as a place for people to undergo training for their souls. In this sense, this world is not totally imaginary. This world is a place where the soul borrows the temporary form of flesh for the sake of self-expression. Be that as it may, a physical body must inevitably enter the path of decline. Therefore, even if you pursue happiness in this world, that will not be a final form of happiness. It is important to pursue happiness that will continue from this world to the next. This is the happiness called "enlightenment." [...]. In short, as long as people are attached to the bodily portion, or the temporary portion of this world, ultimate happiness cannot be achieved. This world is a world of flux in which all things are transient, and nothing is permanent. Human beings cannot remain young and beautiful forever. As we get older, our hair turns white, we get hunched over at the waist, and our faces become wrinkled. Eventually, we become ill and die. Birth, Aging, Illness and Death were unavoidable 2,500 years ago and still are today. [...]. As far as life in this world is concerned, it is important to live, as happily as possible, but after passing a certain point, we should be willing to wind things up. After all, this world is nothing more than a stop on the way to the next world. [...]. Human beings living on this earth must all pass through the gateway of death and experience separations from family and friends. Then, in accordance with our achievements in this world, we will go to the next world, a place where our comrades will be. It is similar to the way in which we progress through junior high school, high school, and finally college, based on our individual academic abilities. Accordingly, it will not do good to regret separations. To the end, it is best to have ingrained the feeling that all things are transient."

4. Physical Factors

As mentioned above, Happy Science theory does not deny that various physical factors contribute to diseases; specifically, almost all modern diseases are caused by what we eat, lack of exercise, and stress. For example, Master Okawa has warned that if we continue to gorge on salty and high-calorie foods while ignoring exercise, then it is only a matter of time before we get sick; he believes that we should begin taking steps in our mid-thirties to avoid developing what are known as "lifestyle diseases" (Okawa, 2008a). He has also pointed out that, if the body becomes ill, the spirit will steadily rot away, resulting in increasingly more discontent and complaints. In short, if the body is ill, the mind too will become ill. As Buddhism has put it: "In this world, the body and mind are united and cannot be divided—they influence another." Therefore, care of the body is extremely important. Proper nutrition, the right amount of exercise, and the appropriate degree of rest are the keys to health (Okawa, 2008c), and are completely compatible with the suggestions of modern medicine (Weil, 2011). Thus, this section will describe various disease-related physical factors such as a lack of exercise, poor nutrition, physical fatigue, poor sleeping habits, and genetic factors.

4.1. Lack of Exercise

For lack of exercise, Master Okawa has recommended that we begin with walking (Okawa, 2008c). In particular, those living in the city often find it difficult to set aside a place and time for walking; in many cases, they only walk when commuting to and from work. However, if they can walk enough, their mental functions will improve. This is a basic form of exercise. We are also recommended to carry a pedometer daily and record in a notebook how many steps are taken during that particular day before going to sleep, and we should weigh ourselves at least once a day and record our body fat ratio. This is important because even at the same weight, if the amount of fat increases, then the amount of muscle conversely declines. Therefore, if we maintain the same weight, but reduce our body fat ratio, then the overall proportion of muscle will increase. Next, we might consider setting aside some money for exercise, because certain forms of exercise (e.g., walking and jogging) that cost nothing are usually not pleasurable and cannot be continued for long. If we spend some money each month, we can visit a gym to work out or swim or go golfing. Of course, people who cannot spend much money should resolve to spend time on their exercising instead. There are a number of forms of exercise that cost nothing but are still pleasurable, such as jumping rope, swinging around a baseball bat, or practicing a golf swing.

4.2. Poor Nutrition

In the case of poor nutrition, both modern medicine and Happy Science suggest that intake of too many calories or too much water or salt can cause disease (Okawa, 2009a). Master Okawa confessed that he lost 12 kg over three months from an initial weight of 72–73 kg. Nowadays, he maintains a weight of 61 kg, which allows him to work with ease. Based on his diet experience, he has recommended suppressing eating behavior and trying to gradually decrease the body weight by 2 kg per month until the desired weight is reached. In addition, he encourages us to inhibit intake of salt by 7 g per day. Intake of too much water is called "president's illness," because such individuals usually drink numerous cups of green tea or coffee during company meetings. Master Okawa has speculated that there is a relationship between intake of too many calories and tumors or warts; specifically, when an individual becomes overweight, the physical body creates tumors in his or her internal organs or warts on the body surface in order to excrete toxins (Okawa, 2011a). Furthermore, if individuals experience aggressive emotions or are possessed by evil spirits (as describe in section 5 ["Mental factors"]) for extended periods, these tumors or warts can become cancerous.

4.3. Physical Fatigue

Master Okawa has emphasized avoiding fatigue, because the majority of people's worries derive from fatigue (Okawa, 2008c). Studies of how the body operates, actually, show that if it is provided with a certain amount of rest, it will be able to work more efficiently. Master Okawa has offered several methods of achieving adequate rest. First, we should take small breaks of about five minutes in order to enjoy an hour of concentration. This is because people cannot usually concentrate for more than an hour at a time and even people with high levels of concentration can only maintain it for two or three hours at most. After three hours, concentration quickly dissipates. Moreover, during lunch breaks, if we have a place, such as a sofa, at the office where one can lie down or relax, we should visit that place without hesitation. Second, we should pay particularly careful attention to resting three specific parts of the body: the waist, legs, and eyes. If we feel pain in the area around the waist—including the hips and the small of the back—then our endurance will subsequently decline. To rest the waist, we must practice stretching our torsos. In addition, the feet must support the body's dozens of kilograms of weight using a very limited surface area. Normally, it is difficult to stand continuously for more than an hour, but most of us tend to stand for several hours at a stretch in various positions. Therefore, it is necessary to have as much time with the weight off our feet as possible. Finally, when the eyes are tired, it affects the brain and stomach, making us nervous. As a result, we can develop a persecution complex for various situations, making it necessary to minimize eyestrain as much as possible. To do so, it is vital to have adequate lighting while reading or performing similar activities, and to keep a distance of twenty centimeters or more between written materials and the eyes. In addition, we should avoid small print as much as possible. It is also important, after using the eyes for a certain length of time, to look away for a little while in order to rest the eyes.

4.4. Poor Sleep Quality

A number of medical studies have shown that poor sleep quality can increase the risk of several types of illnesses (e.g., Redline & Berger, 2014). Despite this, many busy businesspersons regard sleeping as a waste time and sleep as little as possible. Master Okawa has reported on the spiritual significance of sleeping, as follows (Okawa, 2009b): First, sleep is to help us remember that we are truly a spiritual existence. In our sleep, our spiritual body separates from our physical one and returns to the spirit world. Second, sleep supplies us with spiritual energy. Our physical bodies are nourished by intake of food, but our spiritual bodies are nourished by the spiritual energy in the spirit world. Unless we are provided with spiritual energy via sleep, we, without exception, cannot survive. Taken together, we require a sleeping length of about 8 hours on average to ensure our spiritual health.

4.5. Genetic Factors

In addition to the abovementioned physical factors, most diseases involve complex interactions between numerous genes. While an individual may not be born with a disease, he or she can be at high risk of acquiring it; this is called a “genetic susceptibility” or “predisposition.” Genetic susceptibility to a particular disease due to the presence of one or more gene mutations or a combination of alleles need not necessarily be abnormal. However, notably, genes are not “for” bodily attributes: only about 2% of the genome has a known function (Spector, 2013). For decades, the 98% of the genome that did not make protein was dismissed as junk DNA. Some of this junk DNA is now known to regulate the expression of protein-making genes; however, much of it is still dark matter.

For this genetic factor, Master Okawa has suggested that the heredity of spiritual possession might have a greater impact on diseases rather than the physical heredity of genes (Okawa, 2006; Okawa, 2011); that is, evil spirits who possess the parent(s) can be inherited by the children. In the children’s family, the evil spirits produce a hell much like what the parent experienced. After these children grow up, the spirits move on to possess their children. People who are possessed by evil spirits tend to get married to those who are possessed by similar evil spirits. For instance, the daughter of a man with a gambling addiction will often marry a man with a gambling addiction, even though she feels quite upset about her father’s addiction. Evil spirits can thus be repeatedly passed down for countless successive generations.

5. Mental Factors

5.1. Mental Function

Mental factors can cause diseases according to do different theories: “the mind creation theory,” in which the mind actively creates diseases, and “the levee collapse theory” in which the mind passively invites in diseases when its weakest barriers collapse.

5.1.1. The Mind Creation Theory

The subconscious has the power to influence the physical body (Okawa, 2008a). When this power is misapplied, it can lead to self-destruction. Failure to understand this point can result in disease. If, for example, we have negative thoughts within our conscious minds, these thoughts can sink deeply, settling like sediment into the depths of our subconscious. There, they become thought clouds that ultimately lead to disease. This process usually causes cancer. Because cancer is a state in which the body is harboring cells that are actively seeking to destroy the body, it stands to reason that cancer is caused by self-destructive thoughts lodged deep within the mind. Indeed, my meta-analyses of prospective cohort studies (165 studies) indicates that negative psychological factors are associated with higher cancer incidence in initially healthy populations; in addition, poorer survival in patients with diagnosed cancer was found in 330 studies, and higher cancer mortality in 53 studies (Chida et al. 2008).

5.1.2. The Levee Collapse Theory

The levee collapse theory proposes that, when a river overflows its banks, the weakest point of the banks breaks first (Okawa, 2009a). Likewise, when there is an overflow of disease-causing negative thoughts, they seek the weak point in the body and then collapse it. This pathophysiology can cause any illness, including cancer, heart disease, brain disease, vascular disease, and so on. Thereafter, even if the weakest part heals and strengthens, the next weakest part will break when the negative thoughts overflow subsequently. Thus, in the same way that an overflowing river is stopped, the principal cause of the disease (i.e., the weakest point in the body) must be targeted and eliminated. In a broad sense, from the individual to the family levels, small children in stressful household situations perhaps best illustrate the levee collapse theory. Because a child's parents are closest to the child, the state of their minds directly affects the child. Negative thoughts influence the weakest person in a family and make him or her ill (Okawa, 2008b).

5.2. Mental States

As shown below, there are several mental states that can cause illness. These negative states of mind follow the three worldly delusions of Buddhism: greed, anger, and ignorance.

5.2.1. Addiction (Greed)

Greed, or attachment, is considered excessive desire. Although everybody has desires, when these desires become too extreme, they become an "addiction" in medicine. In the Buddhist doctrine, greed generally refers to indulgence in three major excessive desires: feeding, sex, and sleeping. Such desires can lead to metabolic syndrome (or eating disorders), sexual dependency, and laziness (or sleep disorders), respectively. However, addiction also includes alcoholic dependency, drug addiction, workaholism, gamble dependency, shopaholism, and so forth (Okawa, 2006).

In other words, greed or attachment is the desire to be loved by others to an excessive degree. Master Okawa has pointed out that more than half of our suffering comes from wanting to be loved and recognized, but never having that desire completely fulfilled. In other words, we suffer and worry because we are not satisfied with the love we are getting (Okawa, 2008d). This dissatisfaction can lead to hatred (or anger) toward others or self-abasement (i.e., self-pity), as discussed in the next section. Individuals sometimes try to mask their self-abasement by behaving like perfectionists. Among these so-called perfectionists, there are a depressive character, which leads them to becoming easily disheartened (Ben-Shahar, 2009; Okawa, 2013).

5.2.2. Hatred and Anger vs. Self-Abasement (Anger)

Minds that are harshly critical of others or themselves are full of thoughts of "hatred (or anger)" and "self-abasement," respectively. Individuals with an aggressive character and who continuously produce strong feelings of hatred or anger toward others tend to cause those others to get ill. However, in some cases—when these others have "shining" minds without stains—the will of the aggressive individual has no impact on the others. In this case, the anger and hatred doubles back on those who have produced these feelings, causing them to become ill (Okawa, 2009a; Okawa, 2014a).

On the other hand, self-abasement—wherein people excessively criticize themselves—can cause some severe diseases including cancer. Self-abasement is particularly detrimental to those who have a religious character. This is because these people tend to regard themselves as "children of sin" and cannot forgive themselves; specifically, they cannot forgive the various failures and sins that they committed in the past and suffer from mental agony for years. This subsequently leads to disease (Okawa, 2009a).

Column 1 < Stroke and Coronary Heart Disease >

Those who suffer from strokes tend to be quick-tempered and often get hysterical (Okawa, 2011b). They should avoid "blowing their top" by having a peaceful mind. Indeed, outbursts of anger have been reported as a trigger of acute cardiovascular events including stroke (Mostofsky et al. 2014). Moreover, in one of my meta-analytic studies of prospective cohort studies has shown that anger and hostility are associated with increased coronary heart disease (CHD) events in the healthy population studies and with poor prognosis in the CHD population studies (Chida & Steptoe, 2009).

Column 2 < Breast Cancer, Uterine Cancer, and Uterine Myoma >

Cancers of female organs (e.g., breast cancer, uterine cancer, and uterine myoma) usually develop from marital problems (Okawa, 2009a). For instance, in a case where a husband cheats and does not return home, the wife must dissuade him from having an affair—if she is successful, then the marital problem is resolved and it is unlikely that cancer will develop in her. However, if she is not strong enough to sort it out, she can build up regret in her mind, which ultimately leads to breast or uterine cancers. For many women, being unable to dissuade their partners from extramarital affairs, can cause them to contrarily blame their partners. Furthermore, because they tend to criticize their own value as women, the organs specific to women become afflicted with illness. When this happens, the women can actually make their husbands reflect on their own actions through the women's suffering. In line with this suggestion, a recent prospective study has reported that women with breast cancer tend to be more hesitant in expressing their anger compared to healthy women (Bruno et al. 2014).

5.2.3. An Excuse for Unhappiness (Ignorance)

Ignorance, or foolishness, refers to being unaware of how to resolve one's daily problems. People who are ignorant often make many mistakes and thereby create their own suffering. Many people have failed in their relationships with others or in their jobs, and thus find themselves with no other means of escape other than disease. In their unconscious minds, they want to believe that their sins have been dispelled by their sickness and that they are not responsible for their own failures, and thus make themselves sick. Master Okawa explained this phenomenon as follows (pp.70-71 in Okawa, 2008d): "In the majority of cases, people with illnesses have a desire to be ill. They come to love their sickness, because it provides them with an explanation for their unhappy upbringing, unhappy state of life, and even problems in the future. It might sound cruel to say, but their subconscious loves their illnesses. In other cases, ill people sometimes love their illnesses for the sake of someone else in their family. Some people will become sick for reasons of love. For secular love, that is. They believe that they can save someone in their family by being inferior to them, or experiencing more suffering and problems than other family members. Their idea of happiness is of an extremely low level. They believe that other members of the family will experience happiness as long as there is someone else in their family who is unhappy."

In other words, ignorance or foolishness means nescience of the Truth; particularly, it means a lack of spiritual views on life. This lack of perspective can lead to a fear of diseases or death. In addition to the desire to be loved by others, our troubles are caused by fear (Okawa, 2013). The rules of attraction can be said to work contrarily to our feelings (Hill, 2008); that is, we attract to us what we fear. Fear draws to us that which terrifies us in the very depths of our hearts and minds, in the layers of our subconscious. The subconscious, in fact, cannot discern between good and evil in what we feel and think about deep inside our heart, so it draws to us whatever our subconscious finds. Some people have a habit of worrying that they will get sick someday. When such people go to the hospital, and the doctor happens to mention certain symptoms, sometimes their health actually does collapse all of a sudden. These people are drawing what they fear down upon their own heads.

Column 3 < Atopic Dermatitis 1 >

The skin separates the inside of the body from everything outside of it—it acts as a partition between the body and the surrounding world. Thus, skin abnormalities suggest a discontinuity between the inside and outside. The "inside and outside" refer to the "individual's awareness and soul," and their "relationship with others," respectively. With children, inside and outside also refer to what is within the home and what is outside of it. In other words, the skin is the borderline between the "self" and "others" and between the "inside of the household" and the "outside of the household." When there is a problem with this border, then eczema can be the result (Okawa, 2008b). Specifically, eczema comes from a rejection of the outside world. A previous review has shown that psychological interventions including communication skills can significantly improve the symptoms of atopic dermatitis (Chida et al. 2007).

Column 4 < Presbyopia and Ureteral Stones >

From Master Okawa's own life story, parental stress over children's education can cause presbyopia or ureteral stones (Okawa, 2011b). When he was 44 years old, his first child took a school examination. This caused Master Okawa to feel stressed and made it difficult for him to see; however, his eyesight recovered just for one week by his telling his own eyes to read books without glasses. In addition, every time his first child took a large mock examination, Master Okawa suffered from a ureteral stone. Indeed, a medical university's home page has reported that people with highly stressful life experiences are more likely to develop stones than are those who have not had a stressful experience (University of Maryland Medical Center, 2014).

Column 5 < Dementia >

Elderly people who have memories that they do not wish to recall often unconsciously want to weaken those memories as a defense mechanism. This causes them to suffer from brain diseases such as dementia. In many cases, these elderly people do not remember many past events in their lives. In medical research, because the number of patients suffering from dementia has been increasing worldwide, much attention has been paid to the possible causal links of various psychosocial stressors and neurological diseases that cause dementia, such as Alzheimer's disease (Fratiglioni et al. 2004). In addition, as described in more detailed in the next section, Alzheimer's disease is critically tied with possession by evil spirits (Okawa, 2014a).

5.3. Malicious or Evil Spirit Possession

Possession by malicious or evil spirits leads to various illnesses, a fact long been recognized by both Christianity and Islam. For instance, the Qur'an and Islamic theology refer to humans, angels, and jinn as the three beings created by God who are conscious. Jinn are thought to inhabit the unseen world, and can be good, bad, or neutral; furthermore, they may be associated with mental illness (Islam & Campbell, 2012). Bad jinn are akin to the demons of Christianity. Academically, "possession" refers mainly to a phenomenon that is visible to the human eye (e.g., a high amount of aggressiveness from a docile person, hysterical laughter, talking gibberish etc). Master Okawa defined possession in a wider sense: rather than being a phenomenon that everyone is able to see and understand, Master Okawa called possession a state in which a being from the spirit world inhabits a person constantly (or for a limited period), and influences his or her thoughts and actions (Okawa, 2012a). Generally, possession is thought to refer to the taking over of a body by a malicious or evil spirit, but gods can also enter people's bodies. Thus, possession actually refers to the state of being possessed by a spirit, be it good or bad.

According to a spiritual searching by Master Okawa (Okawa, 2012a), the spirits of Hell cannot spend all of their time possessing people on Earth. They will come to Earth when somebody is in a condition suitable for possession, but when this is no longer the case, these spirits cannot stay. After they leave a person on Earth, these evil spirits return to their "domicile" in Hell, which is where they ought to be. Hell is divided into numerous realms, such as the Hell of Hungry Spirits, the Hell of Beasts, the Hell of Lust, the Hell of Strife (Asura Realm), and so on, and most of the spirits return to the particular areas in which they belong. When a person on Earth emits negative thoughts, however, the spirits return to possess and whisper in his or her ear. On the other hand, spirits in the heavenly realm have their own duties in the spirit world. For instance, although guardian spirits must look after their soul siblings living on Earth, they too have their own work and their own lives in the spirit world, so generally they only come to Earth when they feel that their advice is necessary. There are times when spirits can possess those living on Earth and times when they cannot.

5.3.1. Law of Same Wavelength Attraction

One particular aspect of spiritual possession is the "Law of Same Wavelength Attraction " (Okawa, 2012a). While living on Earth, we are three-dimensional beings whose minds are confined in a physical body that belongs to this world. Our mind is the core of our soul, however, meaning that it is always connected with the world that exists beyond this one. The mind can be described as akin to an electromagnet: the frequencies transmitted by the mind—namely, the tone of the mind—are constantly being transmitted to and from the spirit world, and the mind constantly affects this world and vice versa.

There is a vast diversity of signals and messages emanating from all kinds of beings throughout the spirit world. When the wavelength of signals being emanated by a spirit exactly matches that of signals being emanated by somebody on Earth, the spirit and human become attuned to one another. When spirits are in contact in this way or when a spirit is needed on Earth, it is possible for the spirit to visit Earth. Therefore, if somebody is affected by an evil spirit, then the reason lies in that person's mind. This problematic state of mind was described previously in the "Mental states" section (e.g., greed, anger, and ignorance). In contrast, if a person's wavelengths are not in accordance with those of the evil spirit, then that spirit will not be able to visit or possess the person. This is why people must tune their hearts to a completely different channel. The wavelength that people should attune to is that of the high spirits (Okawa, 2008b).

5.3.2. Acupuncture Points and Chakras

During an illness, the physical body part that is damaged often has a damaged spiritual form. One of the reasons for this spiritual body damage is animal spirit possession (Okawa, 2012a). The World Health Organization has reported a number of various acupuncture points in the body (361 points in total), located in areas such as the head, neck, shoulders, back, lower back, and legs, which are used in massage, acupuncture, and moxibustion (WHO, 2008). These acupuncture points coincide with the parts of the body that animal spirits tend to possess (Okawa, 2012a). A spirit can possess a body when there is something to attach itself to. When somebody's blood flow is disrupted or congested in a certain area, spirits are able to latch onto that area. The places where this congestion occurs become prone to fatigue or pain and, looked at spiritually, take on a dark shadow. This is where the spirit can attach itself.

For instance, patients suffering from rheumatism or who say that their feet always feel cold often have a snake spirit wrapped tightly around their legs. Those who suffer from chronic headaches or who are always complaining that their head hurts often have an animal spirit possessing their head; such spirits could be snake spirits wrapped around their heads or fox spirits holding their heads with the front paws. Animal spirit possession is also true for abnormally sore shoulders, chronic pains of the neck, or pains in the small of the back.

According to Eastern medicine, these acupuncture points are interconnected with the chakras through pathways called "principal meridians" within the body, along which Qi flows (Winsneski & Andeerson, 2005). The word *chakra* actually comes from a Sanskrit word meaning *wheel*. Chakras are the openings or pathways by which spiritual or subtle energy* is taken into the body and translated into a form of energy that the body can use at the cellular level. Although different belief systems have slight variations, seven chakras are generally considered to exist. Master Okawa has elucidated these chakras as spiritual organs as follows (Okawa, 2012b). One example of spiritual organs is the brow, which lies between a person's eyebrows. This corresponds to the sixth chakra (*ajna* or third-eye chakra) in Eastern medicine. This brow is a spot where strong willpower, a spiritual function that is extremely creative and positive, can be emitted. The eyes are also spiritual organs. When the spiritual eyes are open, they seem to possess an extra gleam of light inside. When the eyes have attained this gleam, it becomes possible to see spiritual

* Subtle energy is defined as one or more forms of energy, which do not appear to be within the electromagnetic spectrum. Unknown at this time is the interaction or the impact that subtle energies have on measurable electromagnetic forces, nuclear energy and/or atomic bonds, gravitational effects, or mass.

things—you will be able to discern people's auras and spiritual bodies. The nose is another spiritual organ. Those who put their nose to spiritual use can detect evil spirits or when a person is possessed by an evil spirit because the spirits or possessed will appear to emanate a bad smell even when there is no actual smell. The area from the throat to the mouth is used when giving lectures, and this area also emits a large quantity of light. Light comes forth in the form of words, so this area, too, can be said to be a spiritual organ. This might be the same as the fifth chakra (*vishuddhi* or throat chakra) in Eastern medicine. The palm of the hand also possesses a spiritual chakra from which light can be emitted. Healing power often flows from here, and by laying hands on someone, that person can be cured of illness. As long as a person's mind is harmonious, the palm of their hand can emit healing power. The heart is another spiritual organ. The heart is easily influenced by outside emotions and is able to perceive other people's feelings directly. On the other hand, if people develop a strong will, they are able to influence those around them. This is equivalent to the fourth chakra (*anahata* or heart chakra) in Eastern medicine. The *tanden*, which is located in the lower belly, is also a major spiritual center. Harmonizing the mind by maintaining a serene heart and patience is a very important practice in various religions, and the spiritual center of this power to harmonize the mind is found in the *tanden,* which might be called the third chakra (*manipura* or solar plexus/navel chakra) in Eastern medicine. In the area below the stomach are the sex organs. The man has a male organ and testicles while women have female organs and a womb. These are also spiritual organs that emit spiritual power and correspond to the second chakra (*svadhishthana* or sacral chakra). If we practice sexual abstinence, we can build up spiritual power. If this energy is used for benign purposes, it can be a great power to blast away evil spirits or help someone advance towards enlightenment, but if used for malicious purposes, it can be a destructive power.

5.3.3. Possessions by Evil Spirits Including "Ikiryo"

If evil spirit possession continues for an extended period, then the astral body is affected and begins to change. As the astral body changes, the physical body is gradually affected and disease begins to appear (Okawa, 2009c). For instance, when the stomach is possessed by evil spirits, gastric ulcers or stomach cancer are likely to appear. More interestingly, if the evil spirit of a person who died due to a certain illness possesses an individual, that individual will begin to show symptoms of the same illness. When this possession occurs in multiple people within the same family, many will believe it to be due to physical heredity, whereas in actuality it is heredity of spiritual possession (Okawa, 2011c).

Indeed, both departed spirits and the spirits of living people can cause diseases. Spirits of living persons are called *ikiryo* in Japanese, and are considered to be the combination of the thoughts of an individual's own desire and his or her guardian spirit (Okawa, 2011c). As described in section 5.2.2 ("Hatred and anger vs. self-abasement (anger)") of this chapter, if individuals are excessively attached to a certain person and feel aggressive or angry towards that person, their thoughts can cling to the person, eventually making him or her ill. This is akin to a curse.

Column 6 < Cancer 1 >

Cancer is a form of possession (Okawa, 2008c). The root cause can be traced back various types of psychosocial stress. If such stress cannot be reduced, problems arise within an organ's spiritual form, which in turn leads to an abnormality in the physical form. Master Okawa has pointed out a relationship between cancer and possession by dead people in the same family (Okawa, 2014a). Although cancer is considered by many to be a genetic disease, it is actually not related to genetic heredity but heredity of spiritual possession. The reason that people of one family tend to die of cancer is that they are possessed by ancestors who died of cancer in their family tree, which causes them to suffer from the same symptoms that their ancestors did. My meta-analysis of various prospective studies indicated that stress-related factors related to spiritual possession are associated with higher cancer incidence in initially healthy populations and with poorer survival in patients with diagnosed cancer (Chida, 2008).

Column 7 < Rheumatism >

Previous reviews of the effects of stress on rheumatic arthritis and systematic lupus erythematosus suggest that the findings for these disorders coincide with the broader literature including both animal models and clinical studies of other rheumatic disorders (Chida et al. 2005; Hassett & Clauw, 2010). In more spiritual terms, rheumatism is almost exclusively caused by spiritual possession (Okawa, 2008b). It is common for animal spirits (originally humans) to take possession of the lower halves of people's bodies, but when these spirits become completely stuck to their hosts, the hosts will experience chronic chills in the lower body and become unable to move. There are also cases in which these spirits possess people's shoulders and necks.

Column 8 < Common Cold and Influenza >

Master Okawa has described what spreads viruses, such as HIV and those causing influenza and the common cold (Okawa, 2008b; Okawa, 2014a). HIV was discovered during the first half of the 1980s, and it is believed that spirits work through this pathogen—the same spirits that earlier in history spread the plague (i.e., "Black Death") and cholera. After these diseases were eliminated via advances in medical science, the spirits slowly transformed themselves, eventually reappearing as HIV. Likewise, it is possible that the Ebola virus might have developed from plaque and cholera. In this manner, pathogens, too, are influenced by spiritual elements. This is why, no matter how much research is done on treatment methods for existing diseases, new diseases continue to appear in rapid succession. Of course, viruses and bacteria are the pathogens causing these diseases, but they, on their own, are not very harmful. It is only when they are manipulated by spirits that they become highly contagious. In addition, exactly like spiritual possession, spirits can cause colds and influenza. In fact, when autumn arrives and the weather cools down, insects die off. At around that point, colds and influenza begin to become more prevalent. It is believed that the spirits of some dead insects that cannot return to the spirit world become wandering souls and gather into swarms, spreading colds and influenza.

Column 9 < Multiple Personality Disorder and Schizophrenia >

Multiple personality disorder is called "dissociative identity disorder" according to modern medical classifications; interestingly, the current diagnostic criteria such as the Diagnostic and Statistical Manual of Mental Disorders (DSM-5) acknowledge that this disorder is described as spiritual possession in some cultures (American Psychiatric Association, 2013). Master Okawa has explained that many of these cases are actually caused by evil spirits (Okawa, 2012c). When a spirit takes possession of a person, it drives out his or her soul, so the person will seem to take on a completely different personality. A possessing spirit cannot retain control forever, however, so when it tires, it leaves, and the body is taken over by yet another spirit. In this way, as many as five to ten spirits can alternately control a person's body. Sometimes, a person's guardian spirit takes over the body, but in most cases, the person's spiritual energy has become very weak, thereby allowing other spirits to take over.

Moreover, although modern medicine regards schizophrenia as a psychological disorder, it is actually caused by possession by evil spirits (Okawa, 2014b). Indeed, a Turkish medical research group has suggested that, because demonic possession can manifest as various bizarre behaviors resembling those exhibited by people with psychotic disorders with delusions and hallucinations, it is possible that the hallucinations accompanying schizophrenia are illusory; in other words "a false interpretation of a real sensory image formed by demons." (Irmak, 2014). In medicine, electro-convulsive therapy, which involves administering electric shocks to patients, has been employed to treat severe schizophrenia. Master Okawa has compared this therapy to an exorcism (Okawa, 2014b). Specifically, he explained that, when a patient with schizophrenia receives electric shocks, the possessing spirits become surprised or frightened and leave, thereby relieving the patient of his or her symptoms.

For dissociative identity disorder or severe schizophrenia, the cause of individuals' personality change is related to setbacks or a crisis in life (Okawa, 2014b). For instance, it could be the failure of a university entrance examination, the failure of a romance, the bankruptcy of a parent's business, or the death of a relative. In a short, when an individual yields to self-hatred and practices great self-denial, his or her soul wants to leave the body. When this happens, evil spirits can be invited in for possession.

5.3.4. Organ Transplants and Possession

Master Okawa has warned us of the negative aspects of organ transplants (Okawa, 2008c). As described in section 10 ("The organs of spiritual bodies") of Chapter 1, organs are not merely material in nature. Organs in fact have spiritual consciousnesses as well. In particular, the heart is the spiritual center where the intentions and feelings of human beings are concentrated. If the heart is removed from someone's body without their complete understanding or consent, and is subsequently transplanted into another person's body, then part of the heart's spiritual body will be transplanted as well. In this case, spiritual possession takes place, wherein the donor's soul is pulled by his or her own heart into the new body. Because the soul of the donor co-exists with that of the recipient in the recipient's body, we might see rejection reactions or other complications. One of the most popular representative examples was introduced in section 10 of Chapter 1 (Sylvia & Novak, 1997). Of course, there are numerous other cases involving interference and various unfortunate developments that have taken place all over the world (e.g., Pearsall, 1998).

5.3.5. Suicide

Historically, in most religious traditions, suicide has been considered a sin; however, there have been no clear grounds for a prohibition of suicide.

Happy Science research has found that some people do not realize that they are a spiritual being even after they have died (Okawa, 2012a). Master Okawa supposed that some people commit suicide thinking that life will become easier in the spirit world if they die. However, the vast majority of those who commit suicide do not believe in the spirit world. As a result, even after they have arrived in the spirit world, they continue to commit suicide. After a while, they tire of the endless repetition and search for somebody who appears to desire to commit suicide, possess him or her, and they commit suicide together. Numerous seaside cliffs throughout the world are famous for the countless suicides that have occurred there. This is because the spirits of those who have previously committed suicide drag other people to their deaths. They look for someone who is wandering around, deep in worry, possess him or her and make him or her believe that the spirit's emotions are his or her own. Then, the spirit lets the individual commit suicide. People who suffer in this world will find that, after they have died, their suffering will increase tenfold or even a hundredfold after death. In other words, our thoughts in this world will be amplified in the next.

5.4. Karma

The karmic law can be called the "law of cause and effect"; it refers to how the accumulation of previous lives manifests in this life (Okawa, 2008c). For instance, someone might be consistently hurt by others because in a past life he or she hurt other people, or that person might lose his or her sight or have a bad leg because he or she injured someone's eyes or leg, respectively, in a past life. If we think of life as a workbook, the most significant problem contained therein concerns not just what arises in this life but also what happened in past lives. The concept of karma should not be approached solely from the perspective of "merits are rewarded and sins are punished." In other words, diseases caused by karma are not necessarily a punishment. When a person is reborn, he or she chooses the life he or she will live. Since people become enlightened only through experience, certain souls will occasionally choose to have a severe illness. This phenomenon is called the "law of compensation" (Okawa, 2014b) or "cutting down the karma," (Okawa, 2011b), and shows how life plans do not contain only good aspects; that is, plans also include necessary events allowing for the soul to achieve its highest potential. People who plan such lives are well aware of the diseases they will face.

The mechanisms by which karma leads to various diseases are as follows: if the soul is stamped with an experience of deep injury and suffering because of illnesses or accidents causing death in past lives, then such suffering will begin to show in that person's new body (Okawa, 2008c). In many cases, the exterior portion of the spiritual body—the astral body—undergoes various changes, which eventually manifest in the physical body.

5.5. Case Report 4 (Soulmate)

Some psychiatric studies have reported on the concept of "soulmates," which refer to a karmic relationship between eternal reincarnations (e.g., Weiss, 1997). In some cases, this soulmate might be critically related to an illness in the current life. The story of one Happy Science member (Miyako Tsuchimine, Japan; Happy Science, 2010), here described, deals with this theme. Her eldest son and daughter were diagnosed with autism, her second son with Asperger's syndrome, her third son with attention-deficit hyperactivity disorder (ADHD), and her second daughter with pervasive development disorder.

The man she had married left everything about raising children to her and had an unstable income. Her firstborn daughter was slow to start speaking and was not able to hold a coherent conversation until she was five years old. Miyako repeatedly asked her husband to stabilize the family's finances and to help her with raising their daughter, but the telephone continued ringing with the landlord's calls about overdue rent money. Unexpectedly, she became pregnant again and gave birth to her second child. Her newborn son was more difficult to rear than her daughter had been. Even when he was hungry, he did not cry or drink milk. She divorced from her husband before her son turned one.

It was around that time that she encountered Master Okawa's books. She said, "Every page was filled with answers to all the things that I, for so long, had wanted to know. I joined Happy Science and later met a wonderful man there and got married." Her second husband adored her first son and daughter as if they were his own. The year following their marriage, they had a second son, with a third son arriving the year after that. With mountains of laundry to do, messy rooms to clean, and four children to take care of, the days flew by. However, her firstborn son remained unresponsive to their voices and immobile even when he should have been at the age to start crawling. If he became interested in a toy, he would focus on it for hours, "but" she said, "if I took to toy away from him, he'd get so violent that I did not know what to do."

Desperate for clues on how to deal with her children, she attended the Noble Eightfold Path seminar at Nikko Shoja*. During this seminar, while reflecting on her life with her eyes closed, she saw a vision. In this vision, she saw the members of her family together as a family during various different eras. In one era, her eldest son brought her to Buddha; in another era, he protected and led her husband and her away from harm. She was bewildered. "My son, the one I thought of as being so much trouble, is one to whom I owe so much in my past life." She was also connected with her other children, and her family was often born together in past lives. Sometimes they had different relationships, but they were always helping each other. She saw each of her children's faces in her mind and felt so much love for them that she began to cry. Now that she knew that fate had made them family, she was determined to nurture their souls with as much love and care as possible.

When her eldest son entered junior high school, he experienced a much stricter group discipline than what he had experienced in elementary school. He said, "I don't want to go to school. It's difficult for me to do the same things as the others." This was the first time he had ever spoke about how he felt. The teachers and the school counselor thought that he might have some sort of developmental disorder, so she took him to a hospital. After several tests, the doctor told her, "He is not intellectually impaired, but has severe high-functioning autism." The other children exhibited similar symptoms to her eldest son, so she had them all tested. The results were that her eldest daughter also had autism, her second son had Asperger's syndrome, and her third son had ADHD. There was very little understanding of developmental disabilities and much prejudice in her community; people in her neighborhood began to spread rumors just from seeing her take her children to the hospital. However, her husband gently told her, "I don't believe these are disabilities even if that is how they were diagnosed. These are their unique characters. Let's believe in their future." She agreed. "The Lord must be telling me to learn from these difficult circumstances. I should keep faith in Him and move forward." Miyako used to be timid and neurotic, worrying about what others thought or about the prejudices in her community. However, as she learned to love the unique personalities of her children and fight against societal prejudice, she found that she had grown stronger and more caring.

---

* Nikko Shoja: a Happy Science temple in Nikko, Japan.

Column 10 < Cancer 2 >

One of the causes of cancer is karma. For instance, Master Okawa (Okawa, 2014a) has reported on a karma reading of a woman suffering from breast cancer after an operation for uterine cancer; he found that, in a past life, this woman had cut somebody down with a Japanese sword. Thus, she might have been suffering from the same cancer as one of the people she had killed in the past. This is called "cutting down the karma." Master Okawa has explained that, when somebody cuts or kills someone with an edged tool in a past life, his or her karma often causes a type of illness needing surgery. It does not matter whether the people these individuals cut down are good or bad.

Column 11 < Birthmarks and Birth Defects >

A distinctive birthmark, in many instances, closely corresponds with the way in which an individual died in a past life (Okawa, 2008c). Indeed, these marks are located on the same parts of the body where in past lives they were fatally struck by a sword, spear, or arrow. The Division of Perceptual Studies at the University of Virginia has reported that many of karmic birthmarks are not small discolorations (Tucker, 2005). Instead, they are often unusual in shape or size and are puckered or raised rather than flat. Some can be quite dramatic and unusual in appearance. For example, there are several cases in which a small, round birthmark matching a typical bullet entrance wound and a larger, more irregularly shaped birthmark matching a typical exit wound were both present in an individual who had never been shot. Other examples include cases with birthmarks in unusual places, such as wrapped around an ankle, and or deformities such as missing or malformed limbs or digits. In these cases, the birthmarks or birth defects can provide a concrete indication of a connection between the present illness and a past life. More surprisingly, research has indicated that up to a third of cases from India include birthmarks or birth defects that are thought to correspond to wounds from previous lives (Tucker, 2005).

Column 12 < Atopic Dermatitis 2, Asthma, or Bronchitis >

In addition to resulting from human relationships, atopic dermatitis might be due to karma (Okawa, 2008c). There are many cases in which atopic dermatitis can be connected to the way the afflicted person died in a past life. For instance, people who were burned to death might manifest various forms of skin disease or severe atopic dermatitis. Additionally, people who died in fires might have, instead of burning to death, painfully suffocated to death from the smoke. These people may suffer from asthma, bronchitis, or another form of respiratory disease in their current lives.

Column 13 < Phobia >

Psychology has revealed much in the past century about sexual traumas and fears. Nevertheless, without karma readings into past incarnations, we cannot specify the real causes in some phobia cases, such as panic disorder, hydrophobia (fear of water), acrophobia (fear of heights), claustrophobia (fear of enclosed spaces), androphobia (fear of men), and obsessive-compulsive neuroses (Okawa, 2008b; Okawa, 2008c). In this life, the causes can vary, including experience of violence when young or being the victim of sexual abuse. While it is not wrong to say that these are the causes, a deeper investigation of a considerable number of cases has revealed that feelings of terror for specific objects or people can be traced back to past lives (Okawa, 2008b; Okawa, 2008c). For instance, a person who died in a flood in a past life will naturally have a fear of water. Additionally, a person who was killed in a sudden night attack or an individual who was suddenly and indiscriminately cut down in the street during a civil war might continuously suffer, even in this lifetime, from fears of the unknown. Even though it is possible to identify the origins of a fear in this life, according to Happy Science, the root cause of a disease is found farther in the past. In the past-life studies by the Division of Perceptual Studies at the University of Virginia (Tucker, 2005), many subjects showed a phobia related to the mode of death of the previous personality. Indeed, in cases where the previous personality died by unnatural means, more than 35% of the subjects showed phobias related to a previous life. This seemed particularly common for drowning cases (appearing in 31 out of 53 cases). One might speculate that this increased frequency is because drowning victims spend more time in the process of dying than do individuals who are killed in an automobile accident or who are shot to death.

Column 14 < Gender Identity Disorder >

Patients with gender identity disorder (GID) in general show an identification with the opposite sex and discomfort with their own sex. Though there is much research on the topic, its cause is still largely unknown. Some have speculated that sex hormones during pregnancy are involved, but little direct evidence is available to support that. The past life research of the Division of Perceptual Studies at the University of Virginia has reported a number of cases involving a sex change between past lives, wherein the child claims to remember the life of a member of the opposite sex. In these cases, the researchers observed cross-gender behavior. In one series of sex-change cases, 21 out of 34 cases (62%), showed behavior appropriate for the opposite sex (Tucker, 2005). Master Okawa has offered an explanation for GID (Okawa, 2008b), proposing that there are three types of human being: those repeatedly reborn as male; those repeatedly reborn as female; and those reborn as different sexes. In most cases, GID arises when all the soul siblings are female or male but an individual is born as the opposite sex. From a religious standpoint, one cannot consider GID a "disease." It is merely a case of being clearly conscious of one's own sexual nature. When one considers the full range of reincarnations, many people are born alternately as male or female. This is because unless a soul takes on both genders, its life experience is likely to be insufficient.

Column 15 < Abortion >

The problem of abortion (i.e., intentional miscarriage) has arisen because almost all human beings are unaware of the mechanism by which souls are reborn (Okawa, 2008b). Master Okawa has pointed out that Heaven is now in a state of utter confusion because of abortions. Although the various spirits of Heaven are eager to come to Earth, there are cases in which individuals with important plans are aborted. By being aborted while in their mothers' wombs, these souls incur severe wounds. As a result, the next time they consider going to Earth, they are confronted with the fear that they may be aborted again. In addition, it would take about twenty earthly years for the soul to develop, in the spirit world, an adult consciousness. The spirits connected to this individual will therefore have to care for this spiritual child in the spirit world from infancy, up until it can develop its adult consciousness. This is a great setback for the evolution of the soul. Abortion should be avoided whenever possible.

5.6. Teachers for Human Beings

At present, developed countries are excessively wealthy, which has resulted in numerous "diseases of affluence," contempt for others, and vaulting ambitions. However, most people are not even aware that they have become infected with an illness of the mind. Severely sick people and individuals born with disabilities serve as teachers for those individuals infected with these illnesses of the mind; their message is, simply, "how happy one must be to have been born with a sound body or into a well-off family" (Okawa, 2008c).

In such a case, the illness is not caused by karma, but rather intentionally by these unfortunate people to teach others to not act mistakenly or stray from the right path; these people with intentional illnesses also point out mistakes of the mind (i.e, being unaware of how happy one must be to have been born with a sound body or into a well-off family) in others. By showing us that such problems exist, the disabled and unfortunate can provide guidance for others. For example, Helen Keller intentionally chose to be reborn with the double handicap of being deaf and blind, and tried to teach the world something through her disability (Okawa, 2008b). It is for the reason of inspiring others with courage, joy, and a sense of life's purpose that these individuals choose to be born with a physical disability.

Column 16 < Autism, Asperger's Syndrome, and ADHD >

Modern medicine has suggested that autism is a disorder rather than a disease. However, at the same time, it corresponds to problems in the functions of the human body, especially certain areas of the brain. Master Okawa has speculated that doctors are quick to use the label "autism," "Asperger's syndrome," or "ADHD" for anyone whose unusual behavior and actions are troublesome to deal with and end up causing problems for parents and teachers (Okawa, 2008b). However, when we look more closely, we might notice that most people today attempting to make a name for themselves are "unusual." Indeed, some medical researchers have identified famous figures—scientists, artists, politicians, and philosophers—from the past whose behavior suggests they may have had autism, Asperger's syndrome, or ADHD. Furthermore, these disorders were not defined until the mid-20th century (e.g., James, 2005). Thus, Master Okawa has recommended that, if a doctor tells you that your son or daughter has autism, Asperger's syndrome, or ADHD, then you should not let such a diagnosis trouble you. Instead, you should have faith that your child has a strongly individualistic personality. Moreover, he has pointed out that the characteristics of those with Asperger's syndrome overlap in many ways with the features of those who are angels of light (i.e., inhabitants of the seventh or more dimensions). Namely, both are very particular about cleanliness, have strong senses of justice and fairness, and always fight against evil (Okawa, 2008b).

REFERENCES

American Psychiatric Association. (2013). *Diagnostic and Statistical Manual of Mental Disorders Fifth Edition*. New York, NY: American Psychiatric Publishing.

Ben-Shahar, T. (2009). *The Pursuit of Perfect: How to Stop Chasing Perfection and Start Living a Richer, Happier Life*. New York, NY: McGraw-Hill.

Bruno, A., Pandolfo, G., Scimeca, G., Leonardi, V., Cedro, C., Racchiusa, S., Zoccali, R.A., & Muscatello, M.R. (2014). Anger in health, benign breast disease and breast cancer: a prospective case-control study. *In Vivo*, 28, 973-977.

Chida, Y., Sudo, N., & Kubo, C. (2005). Social isolation stress exacerbates autoimmune disease in MRL/*lpr* mice. *Journal of Neuroimmunology*, 158, 138-144.

Chida, Y., Steptoe, A., Hirakawa, N., Sudo, N., & Kubo, C. (2007). The effects of psychological intervention on atopic dermatitis: a systematic review and meta-analysis. *International Archives of Allergy and Immunology*, 144, 1-9.

Chida, Y., Hamer, M., & Steptoe, A. (2008). Do stress-related psychosocial factors contribute to cancer incidence and survival? *Nature Clinical Practice Oncology*, 5, 466-475.

Chida, Y. & Steptoe, A. (2009). The association of anger and hostility with future coronary heart disease. *Journal of the American College of Cardiology*, 53, 936-946.

Fratiglioni, L., Paillard-Borg, S., & Winblad, B. (2004). An active and socially integrated lifestyle in late life might protect against dementia. *Lancet Neurology*, 3, 343-353.

Happy Science (2010). Member Life Experience. In Happy Science (Ed.) *Diversity Happy Science Monthly Issue 199*. Oct, 2010.

Hassett, A.L. & Clauw, D.J. (2010). The role of stress in rheumatic diseases. *Arthritis Research & Therapy*, 12, 123.

Hill, N. (2008). *Napoleon Hill's Golden Rules: The Lost Writings*. New York, NY: Wiley.

Irmak M.K. (2014). Schizophrenia or Possession? *Journal of Religion and Health*, 53,773-777.

Islam, F. & Campbell, R.A. (2012). "Satan has afflicted me!" Jinn-possession and mental illness in the Qur'an. *Journal of Religion and Health*, 53,229-243.

James, I. (2006). *Asperger's Syndrome and High Achievement: Some Very Remarkable People*. London, UK: Jessica Kingsley Publisher.

Kübler-Ross, E. (1997). *The Wheel of Life: A Memoir of Living and Dying*. New York, NY: Scribner.

Mostofsky, E., Penner, E.A., & Mittleman, M.A. (2014). Outbursts of anger as a trigger of acute cardiovascular events: a systematic review and meta-analysis. *European Heart Journal*, 35, 1404-1410.

Okawa, R. (2006). *A Clue for Sorting Out Family Problems*. Tokyo, Japan: Happy Science. (Available only in Japanese and published as the Japanese title of "Kazoku Mondai Kaiketsu no Hinto" in 2006 by Happy Science).

Okawa, R. (2008a). Part III. The Power of Faith is the Key to Good Health. In R. Okawa (Ed.) *Healing Yourself: The True Relationship between Mind and Body* (pp. 187-225). Tokyo, Japan: IRH Press.

Okawa, R. (2008b). Part II. Q&A Effective Advice for Mind and Body. In R. Okawa (Ed.) *Healing Yourself: The True Relationship between Mind and Body* (pp. 75-185). Tokyo, Japan: IRH Press.

Okawa, R. (2008c). Part I. Building a Happy Relationship Between Mind and Body. In R. Okawa (Ed.) *Healing Yourself: The True Relationship between Mind and Body* (pp. 13-80). Tokyo, Japan: IRH Press.

Okawa, R. (2008d). Chapter 2 Becoming Someone Who is Loved. In R. Okawa (Ed.) *My Lover, Cross the Valley of Tears* (pp. 53-77). Tokyo, Japan: Happy Science.

Okawa, R. (2009a). Chapter 3 The Recovery of Health. In R. Okawa (Ed.) *The Way to Definite Health* (pp. 99-153). Tokyo, Japan: IRH Press. (Available only in Japanese and published as the Japanese title of "Chō Zettai Kenkō Hō" in 2009 by IRH Press).

Okawa, R. (2009b). Chapter 2 Coping with Depression. In R. Okawa (Ed.) *The Way to Definite Health* (pp. 69-97). Tokyo, Japan: IRH Press. (Available only in Japanese and published as the Japanese title of "Chō Zettai Kenkō Hō" in 2009 by IRH Press).

Okawa, R. (2009c). Chapter 1 Health and Happiness. In R. Okawa (Ed.) *The Way to Definite Health* (pp. 15-67). Tokyo, Japan: IRH Press. (Available only in Japanese and published as the Japanese title of "Chō Zettai Kenkō Hō" in 2009 by IRH Press).

Okawa, R. (2011a). Chapter 4 Illness Reading (Q&A). In R. Okawa (Ed.) *The Miraculous Way to Overcoming Cancer* (pp. 135-175). Tokyo, Japan: IRH Press. (Available only in Japanese and published with the Japanese title of "Kiseki no Gan Kokufuku Hō" in 2011 by IRH Press).

Okawa, R. (2011b). Chapter 3 The Way to Cancer Disappearance. In R. Okawa (Ed.) *The Miraculous Way to Overcoming Cancer* (pp. 89-134). Tokyo, Japan: IRH Press. (Available only in Japanese and published with the Japanese title of "Kiseki no Gan Kokufuku Hō" in 2011 by IRH Press).

Okawa, R. (2011c). Chapter 2 Miraculous Healing Power. In R. Okawa (Ed.) *The Miraculous Way to Overcoming Cancer* (pp. 51-88). Tokyo, Japan: IRH Press. (Available only in Japanese and published as the Japanese title of "Kiseki no Gan Kokufuku Hō" in 2011 by IRH Press).

Okawa, R. (2012a). Chapter 2 The Principle of Spiritual Possession. In R. Okawa (Ed.) *The Mystical Laws: Transcending the Dimensional Barrier* (pp. 73-135). Tokyo, Japan: IRH Press.

Okawa, R. (2012b). Chapter 4 Occultism as Power. In R. Okawa (Ed.) *The Mystical Laws: Transcending the Dimensional Barrier* (pp. 197-243). Tokyo, Japan: IRH Press.

Okawa, R. (2012c). Chapter 3 The Principle of Channeling. In R. Okawa (Ed.) *The Mystical Laws: Transcending the Dimensional Barrier* (pp. 137-195). Tokyo, Japan: IRH Press.

Okawa, R. (2013). Chapter 2 I Will Never Say Die. In R. Okawa (Ed.) *The Laws of Future* (pp. 69-99). Tokyo, Japan: Happy Science.

Okawa, R. (2014a). Chapter 4 Disease Reading. In R. Okawa (Ed.) *The Healing Power* (pp. 181-228). Tokyo, Japan: IRH Press. (Available only in Japanese and published with the Japanese title of "Za Hīringu Pawā" in 2014 by IRH Press).

Okawa, R. (2014b). Chapter 2 Disease and Karma, About Trouble by Evil Spirits. In R. Okawa (Ed.) *The Healing Power* (pp. 59-123). Tokyo, Japan: IRH Press. (Available only in Japanese and published with the Japanese title of "Za Hīringu Pawā" in 2014 by IRH Press).

Pearsall, P.P. (1998). *Heart's Code.* New York, NY: Broadway.

Redline, S. & Berger, N.A. (2014). *Impact of Sleep and Sleep Disturbances on Obesity and Cancer.* New York, NY: Springer.

Spector, T. (2014). *Identically Different: Why We Can Change Our Genes.* New York, NY: Overlook Books.

Sylvia, C. & Novak, W. (1997). *A Change of Heart.* New York, NY: Little, Brown & Company.

Tucker, JB. (2005). *Life Before Life: A Scientific Investigation of Children's Memories of Previous Lives.* New York, NY: St. Martin's Press.

University of Maryland Medical Center (2014). *Kidney stones.* University of Maryland Medical Center's official home page. Available from:

http://umm.edu/health/medical/reports/articles/kidney-stones. Accessed Feb 26, 2015.

Weil, A. (2011). *Spontaneous Happiness.* New York, NY: Little, Brown and Company.

Weiss, B. (1997). *Only Love is Real: A Story of Soulmates Reunited.* New York, NY: Piatkus Books.

WHO Regional Office for the Western Pacific. (2008). *WHO Standard Acupuncture Point Locations in the Western Pacific Region.* New York, NY: WHO.

Wisneski, L.A. & Anderson, L. (2005). *The Scientific Basis of Integrative Medicine.* Boca Raton, FL: CRC Press.

Chapter 3

Medical Care in Happy Science Medicine

1. Medical Care Is Love

Hippocrates (460–370 BC), a Greek physician and one of the most prominent figures in the history of medicine, declared that "Whenever the art of medicine is loved, there is also a love of humanity." Eastern medicine has also traditionally regarded medical care as a benevolent art. In line with this, the Happy Science doctrine regards medicine as a form of love (Okawa, 2012a).

Master Okawa defined love as follows (page 1 in Okawa, 2011a): "The essence of love is to be found in the soul's desire to be reunited with God from whom we originated. As we live our individual lives with our different personalities, we remember the ultimate parent and wish to go back to the bosom, to return to the one original source. This is the basis of love. It is vital to accept the idea that we all originate from one being. The truth is that all human beings, as well as plants and animals, originate from one single source. In this respect, we can say that love is a feeling of oneness with others. Love is based on the understanding that you and others are not separate but essentially one, and living others is exactly the same as loving yourself. Similarly, when you love others, it means that you love God Himself."

2. Stages of Love

As described above, Happy Science Medicine is based on love, and thus its medical care could be logically composed of the "Stages of Love," an original theory of Happy Science (Okawa, 2011a).

The first stage is *fundamental love*, a basic form of the "love that gives." This is the love between family members or friends. In its broadest form, fundamental love includes the love we have for the community and society as a whole. Fundamental love is a natural feeling, which is why it is the basis of all stages of love. We are all born with the ability to give fundamental love, and we intrinsically know how wonderful this form of love is; we inherently experience happiness through acts related to giving love. If every person could practice this base form of love, our world would transform into Heaven. Literally, it would shift from the third dimension into the fifth dimension in the spirit world, the Realm of Good, because this dimension is regarded as the Realm of the Good, as described in section 7.1 of Chapter 1. Thus, practicing fundamental love is the first step to creating Heaven on Earth.

The second stage in the development of love is *spiritually nurturing love*. Although fundamental love is not easy to put into practice consistently, everyone has an innate potential to exercise it. In contrast, not everyone has the ability to put spiritually nurturing love into practice because it is a love that leads (i.e., love that leads). Spiritually nurturing love is an intellectual and rational type of love. You cannot truly lead others until you have developed the intellect and insight necessary to grasp the actual conditions of current society. Leaders must possess acute powers of reasoning so that they can solve the problems they find. Spiritually nurturing love is the love practiced in the Light Realm, the sixth dimension of Heaven.

The third stage of love is *forgiving love*. People who practice forgiving love have already undergone a transformative spiritual awakening; indeed, many virtuous religious leaders possess forgiving love. It is a love that transcends the dichotomy of good and evil and represents a state of mind completely devoted to one's sacred mission. This state of mind arrives only after an individual has attained a virtue that surpasses intellectual skill: a magnanimous and merciful heart. Those who can exercise forgiving love are inhabitants of the seventh dimension (the Bodhisattvas Realm).

The fourth stage of love is *love incarnate*, which goes beyond the love of one person for another and the status-related love associated with leadership and forgiveness. Love incarnate occurs when a person's very being emanates love. Even the briefest encounter with love incarnate will free you from worries and suffering, awaken you to the Truths, guide you to feel remorse for your mistakes, and return you to the right path. Love incarnate is associated with the giants of history, those who have towered above the rest by serving as lights of the world and becoming the very spirits of their ages (e.g., Albert Einstein <a physicist>, Napoléon Bonaparte <Emperor of France>, and Socrates <Greek philosopher>). This love belongs to those dwelling in the Tathagata Realm, or the eighth dimension.

3. Eightfold Path and Love

As shown in Table 1, Master Okawa has related the stages of love to the eightfold path of Buddhism, which guides individuals towards living righteously as human beings. He has explained that, while the stages of love help us bring our long-term goals (i.e., training the soul) into daily spiritual practice, the eightfold path focuses on daily actions to cultivate discipline (Okawa, 2013a). Thus, in Happy Science medical care, it is necessary to consider not only the stages of love but also the eightfold path.

Table 1. The Relationship between Stages of Love and Eightfold Path

Stages of Love	Fundamental Love		Spiritually Nurturing Love		Forgiving Love		Love Incarnate	
Noble Eightfold Path	Right View	Right Speech	Right Action	Right Livelihood	Right Thought	Right Effort	Right Mindfulness	Right Concentration

In brief, the eightfold path can be described as follows, according to Master Okawa (pp.83-86 in Okawa, 2013b):

[1] "Right View: Did you look at things the way they are, rightly, based on right faith? Did you observe others rightly? Did you treat others with a compassionate heart, in the way that Buddha would treat them? Did you humbly accept His perspective on life and the world?

[2] Right Thought: Did you think rightly? Is your aspiration for enlightenment appropriate? Did you harbor any negative thoughts in your mind, such as greed, anger, and discontent? Did you think badly of others, or bear malice toward them? Did you become arrogant or doubt Buddha's Truths? Did you have any thoughts that went against Buddha's Truths? Did you make right judgments?

[3] Right Speech: Did you speak rightly? Did you use truthful words? Did you say anything that bothers your conscience? Did you hurt others by using abusive words? Did you lie about the level of your enlightenment, or otherwise use false speech? Did you mislead others by using flattery, or cause others distress by speaking in a way that created distrust between them?

[4] Right Action: Did you act rightly? Did you violate any of the precepts for seekers [of the Truths]? Did your hands, legs, or any other part of your physical body commit any crimes, such as murder, assault, and theft? Did you get involved in any sexually immoral acts, such as extramarital affairs, sexual abuse, prostitution, or an obsession with pornography? Did you respect the lives of all living creatures? Did you make generous and sincere offerings of Buddha, Dharma, and Sangha?

[5] Right Livelihood: Did you live rightly, keeping your actions, speech, and thoughts in harmony? Did you become obsessed with alcohol, tobacco, gambling, or drugs? Did you have any complaints about your life, or did you know how to be content? Did you give thanks for all things? Did you make full use of the twenty-four hours that were given to you?

[6] Right Effort: Did you study the teachings of the Truths in the right way? Did your aspiration for enlightenment remain strong? Did you refrain from doing evil? How many seeds of goodness did you plant? Did you make a constant effort to improve yourself?

[7] Right Mindfulness: Were you able to calm your mind to make a right plan to improve your soul and use your life for the creation of Heaven on Earth? Are your prayers for self-realization in accordance with the Will of Buddha, and do they help raise the level of your enlightenment and further refine your character? Do you have a deep understanding of Buddha's Truths? Do you remember the teachings of the Truths correctly?

[8] Right Concentration: Did you regularly take time for right meditation? Did you engage in introspection about the sins you've committed in the past? At the end of the day, did you look back over your day thoroughly? Did you feel gratitude toward your guardian spirit and guiding spirits? Were you able to attain peace of mind through the practice of meditation?"

Table 2. Categorization of Happy Science medical care by Stages of Love

Stages of Love	Fundamental Love		Spiritually Nurturing Love		Forgiving Love		Love Incarnate	
Noble Eightfold Path	Right View	Right Speech	Right Action	Right Livelihood	Right Thought	Right Effort	Right Mindfulness	Right Concentration
Goal of Right Mental States (Target of Wrong Mental States)	Having Spiritual Views of Life (Materialism or Atheism)	Smiling and Expressing Gratitude (Human Relationship Problems)	Developing Problem-Solving Skills, Strategic Withdrawal, or Optimalism (Ignorance)	Healthy Lifestyle (Evil Spirit Possession)	Detach from Greed (Greed) and Forgiveness (Anger and Hatred)	Developing Altruism (Greed)	Positive Willpower (Evil Spirit Possession) and Faith and Prayer (Poor Spiritual Energy)	Meditation (Stress) Collapse of Karma (Disease-Causing Karma)

Taken together, I have categorized Happy Science medical care in this chapter based on the relationship between the stages of love and the eightfold path. Furthermore, the content is arranged according to the purpose of introducing it into clinical settings (Table 2). Note that care must be taken in practicing the stages of love, as there is an ascending level of difficulty as one progresses through the stages; that is, the difficulty in practicing gradually increases from fundamental love (the fourth dimension) to love incarnate (the eighth dimension). Each will be described from the next section according to the stages of love.

4. Fundamental Love

Fundamental love, or the love for one's community and society, can cure illnesses by seeing others from the spiritual views of life (Right View) and by smiling at and expressing gratitude toward others (Right Speech).

4.1. Having Spiritual Views of Life

In treating illness, it is necessary to first consider its meaning. According to Koenig & Shohaib, (2014), "a common belief in Islam is that physical or emotional sickness is a trial allowed by God to help purify the individual, nullify previously committed sins, and provide an opportunity for future rewards, particularly if the sickness and suffering is handled with patience and forbearance" (page 47). Christians, much like Muslims, have various beliefs about how sickness relates to their religion: some believe that God causes sickness, others that God helps people endure it and suffers along with them, and still others believe that illness is God's test, leading to purification and personal refinement and making the individual "more holy" (Koenig & Shohaib, 2014). In line with these religious philosophies, Happy Science proposes that illness helps develop our soul. Master Okawa, through do karma readings, can follow the thread of individuals' rebirths through countless lives across thousands of years; however, going through each of those lives would be a never-ending task. No matter what happened in our past lives, we must embrace the set of problems handed to us in our present life and attempt find the solutions to those problems (Okawa, 2008a). This workbook of problems to be solved in life is different for each person. However, each workbook will be perfectly suited to the study that each individual's soul must undertake.

Thus, we must not flee from our illnesses or avoid the work of identifying the solutions that those illnesses are calling for us to identify. All of us must seek out the significance hidden within the illnesses that we face. Taken together, when we suffer from illness, we first must humbly reflect upon its significance according to a spiritual view of life (i.e., the fact that all human beings reincarnate in this world repeatedly to further their spiritual growth). This is the first point of care in Happy Science Medicine. Master Okawa has indicated that, since the number of people in this world without spiritual views has increased recently, the incidence of diseases that are actually curable is increasing. These diseases cannot be cured due because people are adhering too much to materialism or atheism (Okawa, 2011b). More unfortunately, even after they die from disease, these individuals are likely to wander in Hell because they cannot understand posthumous existence (i.e., the soul).

4.2. Smiling

Since smiling is a sign of love towards other people, we should try to smile as often as possible. Indeed, Master Okawa has suggested that smiling could be a sovereign remedy for cancer (Okawa, 2011c). He has also speculated that, as smiling decreases, the number of illnesses would increase. Smiling is a matter of mental effort and habit. It is very important to give love to others by smiling at them with as much radiance as a sunflower. This mechanism by which smiling helps to cure disease is that those who always smile receive more love, which is thus converted into medicine to alleviate mental and physical illness. A recent 7-year prospective study showed that a sense of humor is associated with increased longevity (Svebak et al. 2010).

4.3. Gratitude

If we wish to avoid contract diseases, Master Okawa has recommended us to appreciate and express gratitude towards others (Okawa, 2009a). Thankful people do not tend to blame, hate, or rebuke others, whereas those who have aggressive characters or blame others are perhaps more likely to suffer from diseases (as described in the detail in the section 5 ["Mental factors"] of Chapter 2). In particular, those who are not grateful to their parents appear to be more likely to suffer from cancer (Okawa, 2011c). Expressing thanks to others can relieve strain in the present, rather aggression-fueled world. When somebody hates or bullies an individual, having a thankful mind can alleviate or turn aside these aggressive thoughts. We should be aware that how a word is expressed affects our fortunes. A series of medical studies have reported that cultivating gratitude helps strengthen people's immune systems, alleviate their aches and pains, lower their blood pressure, engage in more exercise, sleep longer, and wake up more refreshed (Emmons, 2008).

Happy Science Medicine has recommended developing gratitude by conducting a "Love Balance Sheet" (Okawa, 2002). This practical technique is to try to make a mental list of everything that people have done for us and everything we have done for others. It may be surprising to find that, no matter how hard some of us try, we can think of very few occasions when we did anything for others or tried to make another person happy. On the other hand, it can be easy to come up with situations where somebody else went out of their way in order to help us. Things that we did for others that are genuinely good go into the "assets" column whereas things that others did to help us go into the "liabilities" column. When we add them all up, we might deeply regret the way we have lived and understand that we must transform ourselves.

4.4. Case Report 5 (Gratitude)

In the following story, a Happy Science member (Yuko Suffered, Japan; Happy Science 2010a) encountered the truth and not only found solutions to her problems but also obtained renewed appreciation for her family.

She used to have three questions. The first question was about her eyes. She was born in Japan in 1965 with an eye disease of unknown origin. Because of this disease, she gradually started to lose her sight, ultimately becoming completely blind when she was only 23 years old. She asked, "Why did I have to become blind so young?" In a world without light, all she felt was intense anxiety and despair over her future. The second question was about her marriage. After losing her sight, she worked as a telephone operator when she learned about a program that offered people with disabilities a chance to study overseas. She eagerly applied and, at the age of 35, went to study abroad in Canada in 2001. There she met Thilo, who had the same disability; being attracted to his sincere personality, she married him in 2003. However, soon after they began living together, they discovered that it was difficult to communicate with one another, with them being blind and coming from different cultures. She was also very disappointed with her husband's spending habits. Even after they were blessed with a son, Kurtis, Thilo was still carefree with their money. "Don't you care about your family at all?" she asked. The feeling that this marriage was a mistake grew stronger over time and she began to think about divorce. The third question was about their son. Her husband and she had both wished for a child, so they were extremely happy when she became pregnant at 40 years old. He was born healthy and they loved him dearly. However, some people around them had misgivings about their raising a child. These people said that Yuko and Thilo were irresponsible to do so, making her worry if her son was happy being their son. The word "karma" crossed her mind as she thought despondently on her life—of becoming blind, the difficulties with her husband, and now wondering whether it had been the right choice to give birth to her son. She believed that karma was a negative aspect of life, and that she was suffering the consequences of her behavior in a past life. "Am I like a criminal paying for my crimes in jail? Is that my life?" The agony of living grew larger and heavier, threatening to crush her.

She first met Mikiko Shelly, who introduced her to Happy Science, in 2004, when she was still pregnant with her son. Thinking that Yuko might be anxious about giving birth in a foreign country, Mikiko took care of her in many ways [...]. Mikiko told Yuko that she was a believer of Happy Science and lent her audiotapes of Master Okawa's lectures. *Be Infinitely Kind* and *Live in a Time of Light* were some of the lecture tapes Mikiko lent her. Yuko played the tapes without expecting much, but as she listened to the teachings, her worries seemed to disappear one by one, as if they were being peeled away. "Human beings are born thousands of times, each time choosing their parents, environment, and physical conditions. Whatever our state is now in this world, we will all return to being 100% healthy souls when we return to the other world" (Okawa, *Tips to Find Happiness*). When she learned of this spiritual philosophy of life, she could accept being blind as part of her "training." She realized that doing her best in the current circumstances would provide enormous enrichment for her soul. Gone was the guilt she had felt towards her child; in its place, there was only gratitude that he had chosen them as his parents. From the bottom of her heart, she wanted to do all she could to help him fulfill his own mission. To her relief and surprise, the heavy sediment at the bottom of her heart miraculously disappeared and she felt as if a clear blue sky had opened up above her. "In this way, everybody is presented with the problems best suited to their soul. No matter what you are confronted with, it is one that you will be able to solve. In fact, it is one that only you will be able to solve" (Okawa, *Live in a Time of Light*).

Her relationship with her husband, however, had yet to improve. She understood from Master Okawa's teachings that they would be husband and wife in the spirit world, but she still could not help feeling uncomfortable around him. She again consulted with Mikiko, who advised her to find the good points about her husband. Yuko tried this, but despite her best efforts, could only think of four such points, which only made her more disappointed at how few good qualities he had. When Mikiko heard this, she said to Yuko, "Only four? I can think of a lot more! You need to calm your mind and pray to your guardian spirit." Taking Mikiko's advice, Yuko tried again the next day. As she prayed to her guardian spirit, she once more looked upon her husband and the man that he was. Surprisingly, upon doing so, his good points came to her one after another. By the time she was writing the 20th point, she realized that she had been completely engulfed within his love and she broke down sobbing and crying. "Thilo is such a deeply loving person. He was always thinking of me so much. Why didn't I notice?" She awakened to a new sense of love for her husband —it was a lot warmer and deeper than the love she had felt before their marriage. That evening, they sat on the couch and for the first time in a long while they had a talk as husband and wife. She told him what had happened that day: that she had reflected on him while meditating, that she could not stop her tears after coming up with so many great things about him one after another, that she was a fool to not have noticed his love, that she would like to walk together with him from now on, and that she loved him very much. Her husband cried as he listened to her talk. Then she told him, "I would like to study with you at Happy Science, where they teach the most essential things in life." He nodded while still in tears. In September 2007, they, as a family, pledged devotion to the Lord.

5. Spiritually Nurturing Love

Spiritually nurturing love, an intellectual and rational type of love, can cure illness by helping people to correct their lifestyles (Right Livelihood) and utilize intellectual skills and reason to solve problems in everyday life or workplace (Right Action).

5.1. Healthy Lifestyle

As described in Chapter 2, possession by evil spirits can cause several types of disease. In addition to problematic mind states, an unhealthy lifestyle is another major factor in attracting evil spirits. Therefore, it is also important that patients lead a regular and orderly life, and allow their bodies to rest (Okawa, 2012b). Even if people live with a right mind, if they become exhausted, it is difficult for heavenly spirits to approach them. In fact, if they are too tired, evil spirits become attracted to them and find it easier to possess them. Thus, living a healthy lifestyle can protect us from evil spirits. When we are physically exhausted, we should rest, eat nutritiously, and rebuild our body by engaging in exercise. Unless patients regain their health, it may be impossible to get rid of evil influences.

5.2. Developing Problem-Solving Skills

A person who has a pure mind but fails or suffers from disease usually has poor problem-solving skills (Okawa, 2012c). This situation is related to ignorance as described in section 5.2.3 ("Mental states") of Chapter 2. Solving problems is related to wisdom and the ability to function in this world. If there is a problem that cannot be solved, our resulting confusion and worry can cause devils or evil spirits to possess us, thereby causing several types of illnesses. Even if a person is not evil, when a root problem goes unresolved for a long time, possession could be the ultimate result. Experiencing hardship at work or worrying about family is natural, but if we are unable to detach ourselves from it, resolve it, and protect ourselves through reason, evil spirits can delude us on this point and make a small problem much bigger.

Master Okawa has recommended that we use the "Method of Making a List of Our Current Worries" in order to develop problem-solving skills (pp.58-59 in Okawa, 2014a; Okawa, 2009b). "Let us take a huge pair of scissors and cut off the past and future. There is no point in thinking about them now. There is nothing we can do about past mistakes and failures, so just put them aside for the moment. As for the future, it stretches on and on, into next year and the year after next, and once we start thinking about it, we will have far too many worries to deal with, so let's put them aside for the moment as well. For the moment, just create an enclosure around 'present time' and only look at the problems we are currently dealing with. Furthermore, since there are probably a number of problems that we need to face, count to see how many worries we actually have. Of course, there would be not just one, but maybe five or ten. Then, prioritize these problems and resolve them in turn, one at a time. It is also important to sort them into big problems and small problems, in other words, to separate the important issues from the trivial ones. We could also use the principle of fragmenting. This can be explained using the analogy of clearing snow off a roof. The roof cannot be cleared all at once, but we can scoop up small portions of snow with a shovel and gradually clear it all off. With these methods, we can break our current 'enemies' into pieces and get rid of them one at a time."

5.3. Strategic Withdrawals or Optimalism

In some cases, the nature of the work does not match our personality or requires abilities that we do not have, and we are unable to overcome the problems associated with this work. The best way to deal with such a situation is to withdraw (Okawa, 2012c). Such a withdrawal must be strategically planned. If we do not retreat, evil spirits can influence and control us endlessly. For example, we might request that the task be given to somebody more suited to completing it. If the task is too difficult for anybody, it may be better to reassess whether the goals of that task are realistic and discuss this with others. In this way, we might take a step back and break the problem down into small parts that can be accomplished with our abilities.

In other cases, we are setting ourselves too high standards at home or work, often because perfectionism is seen as a laudable quality. However, medical research has indicated that perfectionism has a dark side, causing not just psychological stress (as perfectionists feel considerable pressure to be "perfect"), but also physical harm—irritable bowel disease, insomnia, heart disease, and even early death (Ben-Shahar, 2009). Regarding this point, Master Okawa has pointed out the following (pp.30-31 in Okawa, 2008b).

> "Not only is it important to believe that you are a child of God or a child of Buddha, but it is also necessary to accept the fact that, to a certain degree, human beings are imperfect creatures. As long as you live in this world, you will always have some kind of human imperfection, as a human being living within a physical body. In this world, it is impossible to live as a perfect spiritual existence. You can only live imperfectly since you must live through all kinks of experiences. This may result in failures or setbacks, but they are your opportunities to practice self-reflection and learn. [...]. Rather than striving for perfection all the time, it is important to focus on improvement,

and strive for better rather than best. [...]. The point is, if you blame or criticize yourself to the extent that you lose sleep every night, then consider aiming for eighty percent of perfection; the important thing is that you continue on your path."

In psychology, the constant striving for "better" rather than "best" is referred to as "optimalism" (Ben-Shahar, 2009).

5.4. Case Report 6 (Perfectionism)

In the following story, a Happy Science member (Kazumi Kaneko, Japan; Happy Science, 2011) describes how she, a perfectionist, overcame her breast cancer.

Three years ago, Kazumi felt that something was wrong with her breast, but after a quick search online, she decided that it was just an inflammation. At the time, she was very busy with work so she decided she would see a doctor when she had the time. However, by the time she finally did see a doctor—at which point she could not get out of bed in the morning because she was feeling so dizzy—she was diagnosed with terminal breast cancer. Without treatment, she had only 4 to 5 months to live. The tumor had already grown to 9 cm in the diameter of the tumor and had metastasized to the lymph nodes and bones. It was far past the stage where it could be removed through surgery. She was told she needed to be hospitalized immediately and undergo anticancer drug treatment.

However, listening to her doctor describe the side-effects of the treatment and the worst that could happen, she was uncertain whether she wanted to undergo treatment. Kazumi was a Happy Science believer and had faith that humans are essentially spiritual beings. Looking back, she remembers feeling strange hearing the doctor talk about her body as if it was a material object. "I don't mean to disregard Western medical science, but as someone who believes that 70 to 80% of illnesses are caused by our state of mind, I doubted surgery and medicine alone could get me better." Soon after her diagnosis, Kazumi attended a public lecture by Happy Science founder Master Okawa. The lecture was titled, *The Way to Definite Health*. "The fact that you have cancer means that an energy with intentions of destroying your body is at work [...]. If you have faith in God and can remain cheerful, positive and kind to others [...], if you can keep such a state of mind, then your health problems will certainly make a turn for the better."

Kazumi strongly agreed with the idea that the cancer was of her own making. If that was so, then it was also in her power to cure it. Convinced, she decided not to undergo treatment and only go to the hospital for tests. So began her days of quiet inner examination in the comfort of her home. Most of the day was spent on reflection. Until then, she had been too busy with work to have the time to stop and reflect on herself. "When I thought about it, I had been over-confident in my health. I thought I would never get sick. I also realized that I hadn't been appreciative of the support my family and the people around me had been giving me." In addition to inner self-reflection, she took care of what she ate, eating foods that would increase her immunity, and exercising to build up stamina. She also went to the hospital once a month to get blood tests, CT scans, and ultrasounds.

"Since I was told that I only 4 months to live, I prepared myself to accept the idea of death. It was hard at first, but when I could accept that it is God who decides how long I live, I realized that God had given me life. After that profound realization, I constantly felt overwhelmingly grateful for just being alive." As she filled each day with gratitude, the tests each month showed that her cancer was gradually decreasing in size, and in ten months' time it had completely disappeared. When she received her final test at a separate hospital in the city, a doctor who saw her medical file could not believe that her cancer had really disappeared and asked her to check into the hospital for three days so he could check her thoroughly. They found no trace of the cancer and, with that, Kazumi returned to work. Her cancer has not recurred until this day. "Even after tests started to show that my cancer was receding, I became anxious if I really could be cured. Coincidently, the test results for that month showed the cancer growing again. The road to being fully cured wasn't always smooth sailing. But to be able to accept that I had created my own cancer was a source of great hope for me because that meant that I could also cure it. The most important thing for me was to really believe."

On how she has changed as a person through her self-reflection, she said, "I used to be a bit of a perfectionist. There was a very strong tendency in me to look as the things that were lacking in myself and in others. If I scored an 80 out of a 100, I was the type that got really hung up on the 20 points that I failed to score. I think that was a major source of stress for me. Now I am able to accept my imperfections. I can also tell myself to work with the good aspects I see in others. It's given me greater peace of mind and happiness [...]. I am who I am now because of my illness. My life is a gift given to me, so I want to spend it for the benefit of as many others as possible. I truly believe faith has made me stronger."

6. Forgiving Love

Forgiving love is the love refined through transformative spiritual awakening. This love has more religious significance than do fundamental or spiritually nurturing love, and reflects detachment from worldly desires (Right Thought) and the development of altruism (Right Effort).

6.1. Detaching from Greed

As described in section 5.2 of Chapter 2, there are three major types of worldly desires according to Buddhism: greed, anger, and ignorance. These desires are the main factors contributing to possession by evil spirits. In this section, the means of detaching from greed in this world is described.

In Buddhism, there is a set of principles called the "Seal of Three Laws,"* which are "all conditioned things are impermanent," "all elements are non-substantial" and "*nirvana* is quiescence." These teachings are very effective in detaching from greed (Okawa, 2015). Briefly, the first principle means that everything is impermanent. For instance, we may be attached to our home, our children, or various other things, but like the current of the river, all things flow and pass. It does us no good to be attached to them. All things in this world will break apart and fall into ruin. The second principle indicates that we should let go of our attachments and remind ourselves that, "the only thing we can take back with us to the spirit world is our mind." We should purify our mind, return to the heavenly world and start our new training there. We should rid ourselves of earthy desires in order to return to the pure world. Earthly desires are attachments to this world based on the physical body. While alive, factors such as money, relationships, a big house, a company, and a name may be useful. However, we must forget them all since they become of no concern after we die. Finally, the third principle dictates that we must understand that the higher realms in the Real World can only be reached by letting go of all worldly attachments; we obtain the greatest happiness in that world.

---

* The Seal of Three Laws (the central principles of Buddhism) is as follows: "All conditioned things are impermanent," which dictates that one should let go of attachments since all things change and pass; "all elements are non-substantial," which dictates that all things are void and non-substantial, and is based on the thought that all phenomena in this world are temporary and that the spiritual world is, in fact, the Real World; and "nirvana is quiescence," which dictates that the state of mind attuned to the higher realms of the Real World is letting go of all worldly attachments. This last teaching is the state of becoming enlightened. All followers of Shakyamuni Buddhism aim to reach this state.

A particular notion in Buddhism is the "Notion of Uncleanness," which suggests that we detach ourselves from excessive sexual desire or lust (Okawa, 1993). Our strong desire for the bodies of others is due to our erroneous conception that they are clean when, in reality, they are unclean. Once we understand the filthy nature of the body, there is no basis for attachment. By holding to the notion of uncleanness, we imagine that others' bodies are filled with countless unclean, unpleasant substances so that they seem to be no more than filth-producing factories. When meditation on this is done well, it can reduce our sexual desire.

6.2. Forgiveness

Forgiveness is a spiritual practice and has been taught by numerous other spiritual teachers, such as Jesus and the Buddha. On this point, Master Okawa has declared the following (pp.31-34 in Okawa, 2014b):

> "Two thousand years ago, I sent Jesus, my spiritual son. But a lot of people killed him. So his spiritual father, himself, came here 2,000 years later. This is the last chance for you. I came here to show that I love you. I have been loving you, and I love you all. Everybody. And I forgive you all. I just want to forgive you all. I have the power to forgive you. Love is forgiveness. A man who can forgive others has a key to love others. Forgiveness is very, very important nowadays [...]. You have many setbacks and sufferings. But bounce back, stand up, and be brave and fight again, because you are loved. You are loved. Be courageous and never forget that you are asked to love God or Buddha. God or Buddha also loves you. Some of you may ask me, 'How many times may I forgive other people, my bad husband or my bad wife?' Someone may ask me. But I'll answer, 'More than 1,000 times, forgive him or her.' More than 1,000. Not one, two, or three. That's the key to Heaven. Heaven is not so far. It's near here. It's at your hand. Please forgive others. Then you'll be in Heaven now."

Since we, as human beings, are not a perfect existence, it is better that we do not lie too much. Numerous people have claimed, "I'm absolutely correct. You're wrong!" and continue to say this for ten years. However, being persistent in this way is evil. Even though the person being blamed might be actually in the wrong, continuing to blame him or her makes the blamers in the wrong. Therefore, if the blamed does not apologize, then the blamers must apologize first. There are numerous diseases that can be cured by forgiveness

(Okawa, 2009a). Recent medical research has confirmed that forgiveness can lead to healthier relationships; greater spiritual and psychological well-being; less anxiety, stress, and hostility; lower blood pressure; fewer symptoms of depression; stronger immune system; and improved heart health (e.g., McCullough, 2008).

6.3. Developing Altruism

Altruism refers to acts to promote another's welfare, even at a risk or cost to ourselves. Though some believe that humans are fundamentally self-interested, recent medical research suggests otherwise: for instance, people's first impulse is to cooperate rather than compete, and toddlers spontaneously help people in need out of a genuine concern for their welfare. Even non-human primates display altruism. Altruistic emotions and behaviors are associated with greater well-being, physical health, and longevity (Post, 2007). Master Okawa has explained about the relationships between altruism and the healing power of Heaven (Okawa, 2008c). Healing light and healing power found in the heavenly world pours freely down onto those who believe and who make honest efforts to move forward in life. The principle is the same as a teacher showing favoritism to young students: If a teacher believes certain students to be more adorable than the other students, then it stands to reason that these students will receive more help from the teacher when needed. Thus, it is incumbent upon individuals to become "adorable children" in the eyes of God. We must live our life in a way that will be pleasing to God, and will cause Him to love us. Moreover, the most important thing in this regard is to be humble, love others, and be kind. Altruistic emotions and behaviors can cure our diseases through the healing power of Heaven.

In terms of developing altruism, there is little help derived from mere altruistic emotion or thinking—putting altruism into practice is absolutely necessary. In other words, to be truly altruistic, concrete efforts must be made. A typical obstacle to taking altruistic or courageous action is the fear of failure (Okawa, 2014c). However, according to Master Okawa, the only thing we should truly fear is fear itself. We must be wary of any fears and insecurities lurking in our mind, and fight them with all our might. Most of our fears and worries are simply the result of inexperience or of not knowing what lies ahead. Master Okawa has taught how to conquer fear (Okawa, 2014c): namely, challenge ourselves to do what we fear the most. Our fears will vanish the moment we face and decide to fight them. Whether we fail or succeed in that fight, the substance of that fear will disappear, and we will be left with only valuable experiences. One of these experiences is that we will have conquered our fear. Another is the feeling of being unsuccessful at a colossal challenge. These feelings will give us a thirst for growth that propels us forward. Conquering these feelings through countless failures will gradually help our altruism mature.

7. Love Incarnate

Love incarnate frees us from worries and suffering, awakens us to the Truths, guides us to feel remorse for our mistakes, and returns us to the right path, through Right Mindfulness and Right Concentration.

7.1. Positive Willpower

Willpower is defined as the ability to resist short-term temptations to meet long-term goals. Recent medical research has found that this ability correlates with higher grade-point averages, higher self-esteem, less binge eating and alcohol abuse, and better social skills (e.g., Baumeister & Tierney, 2011). Master Okawa considers willpower as the power to prevent our bodies from being possessed by evil spirits (Okawa, 2012b). He has recommended that in order to develop willpower, we must suppress as many problematic activities (e.g., drinking alcohol) as possible while putting our hearts into our work or study (Okawa, 2006a).

The key point of developing willpower is the direction of thought: willpower is bright, affirmative, hopeful, and optimistic. However, patients tend to have gloomy, negative, hopeless, or pessimistic thinking patterns. Importantly, human beings reflect the image they hold of themselves (Okawa, 2008d). When we feel that our minds are about to be overtaken by negativity, we must attempt to counter it with our own optimistic energy. It is seemingly impossible for people to hold two contradictory thoughts in their minds simultaneously. People cannot laugh while they talk about something sad, and cannot cry while they are talking about something enjoyable. Indeed, optimism reportedly significantly influences mental and physical well-being via the promotion of a healthy lifestyle as well as adaptive behaviors and cognitive responses associated with greater flexibility, problem-solving skills, and more efficient elaboration of negative information (Conversano et al. 2010).

Regarding the how willpower can be used to change the effects of past events and thoughts of the future, Master Okawa has mentioned the following (page 106 in Okawa, 2008a).

> "If you search your past for the reasons you cannot be happy, you will find any numbers of causes. However, everything can also be a "seed of happiness." Exploring your past and discovering the cause that has made you the way you are today is one method that will give you guidance. Still, the fact is that, if you change yourself right now, then everything in the past will come to appear differently. The past of this life can change, but you can also consider unhappiness in a past life as the seed for your happiness in this present life. It is true that you can go back that far in time to turn your life around. Please have sufficient fortitude to do just that. If we can change the past, then changing the future is very simple."

7.2. Faith and Prayer

Master Okawa has affirmed that "the best medication is Faith" (Okawa, 2011c). Furthermore, the New Testament tells us that Jesus was able to raise people from the dead. For instance, when Jesus came to the tomb of Lazarus and said, "Lazarus, come out!" Lazarus, still wrapped in linen, arose from the slab and came out of the tomb, alive (John 11:1-44). Jesus made the blind see, and made the physically disabled able to walk again. He transformed wine into water. He multiplied loaves and fishes, and then fed a crowd of thousands. Master Okawa has confirmed that these events truly did occur, but we cannot recreate them today. This is because so many people, even Christians, have lost their power to believe (Okawa, 2008c). Medical science has recently learned that a countless number of illnesses are ultimately caused by problems with the immune system. Master Okawa has explained that immunity can actually be boosted through the power of belief and faith. He says that by believing daily that we can act as bodhisattvas in service of God, our entire body will become filled with a powerful surge of positive thoughts. Eventually these thoughts will soak deeply into all of our body's cells and increase our immunity. Boosting our immunity can allow us to win our fight against cancer (Okawa, 2008c).

Considering that, as described in Chapter 1, we are connected not only with guardian and guiding spirits but even with God through the universal unconscious, belief in God can be considered to be almost the same as positive autosuggestion, usually called the placebo effect in medicine. The placebo effect was ranked number one on a list of scientific anomalies that cannot be currently explained with scientific knowledge (Beauregard, 2012). It seems that the more firmly we believe in a particular treatment—whether it be a sugar pill, an injection of salt water, a shaman's curse, or a government-approved medication—the more likely it is that the treatment will succeed. Master Okawa has recommended that we do not take doctors' pronouncements as law—namely, no matter how much our doctor claims that we will never recover or that we will have to continue taking medicine until we die, we must firmly resist negative thinking and affirm to ourselves that we are a child of God and have the power to heal ourselves (Okawa, 2008c). This is called "affirmation" in psychology and is a very powerful method of directing our unconsciousness toward a healthy outcome.

Prayer can be seen as a form of thought transmission, and is received and responded to by the guiding spirits in the spirit world. When one prays, a response is given by the guiding spirits of one's religious affiliation. For example, Christian prayers are heard by Christian guiding spirits. Thus, it can be said that spiritual affiliation is one of the conditions for prayer to be effective. Spiritual affiliation is defined by one's faith. In the same way, Happy Science is blessed by a large number of guiding spirits who provide support and guidance to Happy Science believers. It is debatable whether prayers made by nonbelievers have any effect. Certain spirits may recognize prayers made by nonbelievers, but it is uncertain whether they would ever respond and what type of spirits could be expected to respond. Together with the Happy Science doctrine, my research group has proposed in a published paper the following five theological factors of effective prayer: (1) strength of faith, (2) a becalmed state of mind, (3) readiness to pursue self-help measures, (4) a wish likely to be approved by guiding spirits, and (5) a positive spiritual environment (Kurokawa et al. 2015).

7.3. Case Report 7 (Faith and Prayer)

In the following Happy Science member story (Kikue Shimokawa, Japan; Happy Science, 2010b), Kikue describes how through belief in El Cantare and use of prayer, she recovered from a severe traffic accident.

When she decided to visit Tokushima Prefecture in 2006 with her husband, she had never imagined that this "vacation" would forever change her life. She was chatting happily with her husband about visiting the famous Naruto whirlpools when something struck the car. The windshield shattered and the glass flew onto her. Out of the corner of her eye, she dimly saw her husband hunched over the steering wheel. Although she tried to get out of the car, her body would not move. She soon lost consciousness.

She had fractured her right pelvis and broke six ribs in eight places, and blood had accumulated in her lungs. She had also fractured her left knee and her pubic bone. The injuries were so severe that her chance of surviving the accident had been less than 2%. The doctor told her, "You have suffered almost six people's worth of injuries to yourself." She was incredibly lucky to have survived. While she has almost no memory of the accident, she remembers a dream. Master Ryuho Okawa appeared to her in the dream and said, "I will take care of you in Tokushima for a while…" The feeling was real even after she awoke; she believed that this accident would become a huge turning point in her life. However, after regaining consciousness, reality sank in and she fell into a state of despair from the pain and shock. It takes mere seconds for an accident to rob an individual of his or her own body's freedom, and she was not prepared for it. The more people offered her kindness, the more miserable tears welled up in her eyes. "I will never be able to live a normal life or go back to my workplace again. My dream of someday managing a company is gone," she thought. Completely bedridden, she was always thinking of a time when she was healthy and busy. Until the accident, she had been working as an engineer for a global electronics company. She had devoted herself to developing sensors for digital cameras; she had obtained many patents and had won the company's highest award for inventions twice as well as the National Invention Award. Despite her success, she never forgot the people whose work had made it possible for her to pursue her passion.

The accident shattered everything. She had always believed that her job was all that mattered, and without it her existence was meaningless. She had worked a busy schedule in a world where time was of the essence, but now she was just lying in a hospital bed trying to survive. The surgery she needed to undergo would be very risky; if it did not go well, she could lose her life. The day before the surgery, she prepared for the possibility that this could be the last time she and her husband would ever see each other. "I'll make it out alive." Although that was how she felt, she found herself telling her husband, "Let's be husband and wife again in our next life and even in the life after…" Tears rolled down her cheeks as they said goodbye. The next day, she was taken to surgery. Many of her friends prayed for her recovery. After eight long hours, the surgery was a success. She said, "I am still alive. The Lord is keeping me alive! I still have a mission to fulfill in this life…" Tears flowed as she felt the gratitude of having been given life well up within her. […].

Rehab, however, was punishing. Praying in tears, she asked why God had given her such a difficult ordeal. What was she supposed to learn from this accident? Still crying, she recited *The Dharma of the Right Mind* (refer to Chapter 1). It calmed her and made her feel that she could face another day of rehab. It helped her think, "It's okay to take baby steps; there's no reason to get impatient. I am alive, and it is a blessing to be alive." With rehabilitation, encouragement from countless people, and the power of prayer, her body recovered at a speed that amazed her doctor. After four months, she was finally discharged from the hospital. Looking back, she says, "The accident was an awakening for me. I thought the value of my existence came from the results at work, but all I could do while at the hospital was simply exist." Compared to how she used to think, she says that she has changed greatly. When she was in the depths of sorrow or agony, she felt warm encouragement from many and the love of the Lord. "When I realized that the Lord loves everyone, that he loved me even in my desperate situation, that was when I felt as if I understood true faith." While in the hospital, she often found herself giving advice to friends. Even when she was immobile, she could still smile. "People can give love under any situation," she says. Nowadays, she is studying consulting and her dream is to contribute to her local community.

7.4. Meditation

Meditation is nothing more than directed concentration. One of the main components of meditation is breathing. Medical research has provided considerable evidence that breathing and emotion have a reciprocal relationship: emotional states can affect respiratory rate, depth, and pattern, while voluntarily changing the pattern of breath can account for at least 40% of the variance in feelings of anger, fear, joy, and sadness (Gerbarg et al. 2014). Breathing is controlled by both voluntary and involuntary mechanisms with complex feedback involving the autonomic nervous system, brain stem nuclei, limbic system, cerebral cortex, and neuroendocrine system (Gerbarg et al. 2014). In particular, there are three key benefits of "breathwork" that link the body with the mind and the conscious with the unconscious (Weil, 2011). The first is that breathwork activates the autonomic nervous system and makes it possible for people to influence their own cardiovascular, digestive, and other bodily functions ordinarily beyond conscious control. Second, it is a way to calm the restless mind, facilitating focused attention and meditation. Third, it promotes spiritual development and wellbeing. The simple rules of breathwork are as follows: (1) put our attention on the breath whenever possible; (2) whenever possible, try to make our breathing deeper, slower, quieter, and more regular; (3) let our belly expand outward when we inhale; and (4) to deepen breathing, practice exhaling more air at the end of each breath.

Master Okawa has speculated that psychological stress can facilitate the development of numerous illnesses (Okawa, 2009a) and recommended that we meditate using both breathwork and self-imaging. In particular, he has suggested a special form of meditation for repelling numerous types of diseases (Okawa, 2014d) wherein we try to imagine that our real nature is the spiritual body. Gradually, we come to believe that the spiritual body is our center rather than the physical body. Furthermore, we should conduct a type of meditation before sleep every night in which we imagine the spiritual body as a perfect golden ball. The golden ball is a symbol of "perfection and faultlessness." Although we are at first humans, when we ascend into Heaven, we change into a luminous golden energy resembling a golden ball. This is our true form. Master Okawa has called this form of meditation, the "Self-image Meditation as a Golden Ball." In addition, those who are always thinking negatively should rid themselves of all worldly thoughts in meditation (Okawa, 2006b). At first, we cannot practice meditation without aid for even five minutes. Therefore, we might concentrate on some quiet meditation music or natural sounds such as the sounds of streams, the wind, birdcalls, or waterfalls.

7.5. Collapse of Karma

As described in section 4 of Chapter 1, PLT, a type of hypnotherapy, has been employed as a clinical tool in exploring patients' recollections of past lives, thereby deepening their self-understanding and awareness of current problems and helping to find the key to healing current diseases (Weiss, 1996). Master Okawa has called this a "collapse of karma." He has also pointed out some problems with PLT (Okawa, 2014e). First, the percentage of those who can be hypnotized by PLT is perhaps very low (about 4–10%). Second, patients' stories derived from PLT do not show experiences in Hell. Third, the lives in between our incarnations on Earth do not concretely exhibit the lives of the other world (refer to section 7 of Chapter 1). Finally, there are no clear criteria to distinguish possessing spirits from past lives. A collapse of karma means that, immediately when we understand the reason behind our current diseases by looking into a past life, our diseases disappear at once. In a more religious sense, the collapse of karma corresponds to how self-reflection can cure diseases by grasping the pattern of our souls through deep meditation and identifying its causal association with our diseases. Notably, no matter what happened in our past lives, we must embrace the set of problems handed to us in our present life, and make an effort to find the answers to those problems and questions (Okawa, 2008a).

REFERENCES

Baumeiseter, R.F. & Tierney, J. (2011). *Willpower: Rediscovering the Greatest Human Strength*. London, UK: Penguin Press.

Beauregard, M. (2012). *Brain Wars: The Scientific Battle Over the Existence of the Mind and the Proof That Change the Way We Live Our Lives*. New York, NY: HarperOne.

Ben-Shahar, T. (2009). *The Pursuit of Perfect: How to Stop Chasing Perfection and Start Living a Richer, Happier Life*. New York, NY: McGraw-Hill.

Conversano, C., Rotondo, A., Lensi, E., Vista, O.D., Arpone, F., & Antonio, M. (2010). Optimism and its impact on mental and physical well-being. *Clinical Practice & Epidemiology in Mental Health*, 6, 25-29.

Emmons, R. (2008). *Thanks!: How Practicing Gratitude Can Make You Happier.* New York, NY: Mariner Books.

Gerbarg, P.L., Gootjes, L., & Brown, R.P. (2014). Chapter 12 Mind-Body Practices and the Neuro-psychology of Wellbeing. In C. Kim-Prieto (Ed.) *Religion and Spirituality Across Cultures* (pp. 227-246). New York, NY: Springer.

Happy Science (2010a). Member Life Experience. In Happy Science (Ed.) *Love Happy Science Monthly Issue 200.* Nov, 2010.

Happy Science (2010b). Member Life Experience. In Happy Science (Ed.) *Miracles Happy Science Monthly Issue 198.* Sep, 2010.

Happy Science (2011). Member Life Experience. In Happy Science (Ed.) *Healing Happy Science Monthly Issue 207.* Jun, 2011.

Koenig, H.G. & Shohaib, S.A. (2014). *Health and Well-Being in Islamic Societies: Background, Research, and Applications.* New York, NY: Springer.

Kurokawa, H., Matsumoto, Y., Imai, J., Anderson, T.S., & Chida, Y. (2015). Chapter 8 The Curative Power of Prayer: Happy Science Doctrine and The Theoretical and Theological Base for Prayer-based Health Interventions. In A.M. Columbus (Ed.) *Advances in Psychology Research Volume 104* (pp.129-154). New York, NY: Nova Science Publishers Inc.

McCullough, M. (2008). *Beyond Revenge: The Evolution of the Forgiveness Instinct.* New York, NY: Jossey-Bass.

Okawa, R. (1993). Chapter 4 Five Approaches to Meditation. In R. Okawa (Ed.) *Buddha Silence: The Secret Doctrine* (pp. 127-158). Tokyo, Japan: IRH Press. (Available only in Japanese and published with the Japanese title of "Chinmoku no Butta" in 1993 by IRH Press).

Okawa, R. (2002). *Love, Nurture, and Forgive: A Handbook to Add a New Richness to Your Life*. Brooklyn, NY: Lantern Books.

Okawa, R. (2006a). *A Clue for Sorting Out Family Problems.* Tokyo, Japan: Happy Science. (Available only in Japanese and published with the Japanese title of "Kazoku Mondai Kaiketsu no Hinto" in 2006 by Happy Science).

Okawa, R. (2006b). Chapter 1 Try to Praise Oneself More Often. In R. Okawa (Ed.) *The Laws of Hope* (pp. 29-100). Tokyo, Japan: IRH Press. (Available only in Japanese and published with the Japanese title of "Kibō no Hō" in 2006 by IRH Press).

Okawa, R. (2008a). Part II. Q&A Effective Advice for Mind and Body. In R. Okawa (Ed.) *Healing Yourself: The True Relationship between Mind and Body* (pp. 75-185). Tokyo, Japan: IRH Press.

Okawa, R. (2008b). Part 2. 7 Accept Your Imperfections. In R. Okawa (Ed.) *"I'm Fine" Spirit: How to Get Through Tough Times* (pp. 30-32). Tokyo, Japan: Happy Science.

Okawa, R. (2008c). Part III. The Power of Faith is the Key to Good Health. In R. Okawa (Ed.) *Healing Yourself: The True Relationship between Mind and Body* (pp. 187-225). Tokyo, Japan: IRH Press.

Okawa, R. (2008d). 26 Get Through Tough Times With "I'm Fine" Spirit. In R. Okawa (Ed.) *"I'm Fine" Spirit: How to Get Through Tough Times* (pp. 114-117). Tokyo, Japan: IRH Press.

Okawa, R. (2009a). Chapter 1 Health and Happiness. In R. Okawa (Ed.) *The Way to Definite Health* (pp. 15-67). Tokyo, Japan: IRH Press. (Available only in Japanese and published with the Japanese title of "Chō Zettai Kenkō Hō" in 2009 by IRH Press).

Okawa, R. (2009b). Chapter 2 Coping with Depression. In R. Okawa (Ed.) *The Way to Definite Health* (pp. 69-97). Tokyo, Japan: IRH Press. (Available only in Japanese and published with the Japanese title of "Chō Zettai Kenkō Hō" in 2009 by IRH Press).

Okawa, R. (2011a). *The Origin of Love: On the Beauty of Compassion*. Brooklyn, NY: Lantern Books.

Okawa, R. (2011b). Chapter 2 Miraculous Healing Power. In R. Okawa (Ed.) *The Miraculous Way to Overcoming Cancer* (pp. 51-88). Tokyo, Japan: IRH Press. (Available only in Japanese and published with the Japanese title of "Kiseki no Gan Kokufuku Hō" in 2011 by IRH Press).

Okawa, R. (2011c). Chapter 3 The Way to Cancer Disappearance. In R. Okawa (Ed.) *The Miraculous Way to Overcoming Cancer* (pp. 89-134). Tokyo, Japan: IRH Press. (Available only in Japanese and published with the Japanese title of "Kiseki no Gan Kokufuku Hō" in 2011 by IRH Press).

Okawa, R. (2012a). Chapter 6 The World of the Ninth Dimension. In R. Okawa (Ed.) *The Nine Dimensions: Unveiling the Laws of Eternity* (pp. 137-159). Tokyo, Japan: IRH Press.

Okawa, R. (2012b). Chapter 2 The Principle of Spiritual Possession. In R. Okawa (Ed.) *The Mystical Laws: Transcending the Dimensional Barrier* (pp. 73-135). Tokyo, Japan: IRH Press.

Okawa, R. (2012c). *The Modern Day Exorcist*. Tokyo, Japan: Happy Science.

Okawa, R. (2013a). Chapter 3 The River of God's Love. In R. Okawa (Ed.) *The Laws of the Sun: One Source, One Planet, One People* (pp. 87-120). Tokyo, Japan: IRH Press.

Okawa, R. (2013b). Chapter 2 Buddha's Truths Speak. In R. Okawa (Ed.) *The Laws of the Sun: One Source, One Planet, One People* (pp. 54-86). Tokyo, Japan: IRH Press.

Okawa, R. (2014a). Chapter 1 How to Overcome Slumps. In R. Okawa (Ed.) *The Laws of Perseverance: Reversing Your Common Sense* (pp. 19-74). Tokyo, Japan: IRH Press.

Okawa, R. (2014b). *Be Positive*. Tokyo, Japan: IRH Press.

Okawa, R. (2014c). Chapter 5 Magnifying Your Courage a Hundredfold. In R. Okawa (Ed.) *Think Big: Be Positive and Be Brave to Achieve Your Dreams!* (pp. 121-141). Tokyo, Japan: IRH Press.

Okawa, R. (2014d). Chapter 1 The Mental Power of Curing Disease. In R. Okawa (Ed.) *The Healing Power* (pp. 17-57). Tokyo, Japan: IRH Press. (Available only in Japanese and published with the Japanese title of "Za Hīringu Pawā" in 2014 by IRH Press).

Okawa, R. (2014e). Chapter 2 Disease and Karma, About Trouble by Evil Spirits. In R. Okawa (Ed.) *The Healing Power* (pp. 59-123). Tokyo,

Japan: IRH Press. (Available only in Japanese and published with the Japanese title of "Za Hīringu Pawā" in 2014 by IRH Press).

Okawa, R. (2015). Question 1 How to Increase the Power to Exorcise Evil Spirits. In R. Okawa (Ed.) *Basics of Exorcism: How to Protect You and Your Family from Evil Spirits* (pp. 15-33). Tokyo, Japan: IRH Press.

Post, S.G. (2007). *Altruism and Health: Perspectives from Empirical Research*. New York, NY: Oxford University Press.

Svebak, S., Romundstad, S., & Holmen, J. (2010). A 7-year prospective study of sense of humor and mortality in an adult county population: the Hunt-2 study. *International Journal of Psychiatry in Medicine*, 40, 125-146.

Weil, A. (2011). Chapter 6 Optimizing Emotional Will-Being by Retraining and Caring for the Mind. In R. Okawa (Ed.) *Spontaneous Happiness* (pp. 201-263). New York, NY: Little, Brown & Company.

Weiss, B. (1996). *Many Lives, Many Masters: The True Story of a Prominent Psychiatrist, His Young Patient, and the Past Life Therapy That Changed Both Their Lives*. New York, NY: Grand Central Publishing.

INDEX

A

abortion, 44
acupuncture points, 34
addiction, 28
ADHD, 40, 45
affirmation, 70
alcoholic dependency, 29
altruism, 67
Alzheimer's disease, 32
amyotrophic lateral sclerosis, 22
anger, 29
Asperger's syndrome, 40, 45
asthma, 43
astral body, 14, 40
atopic dermatitis, 31, 42
autism, 45
autosuggestion, 69

B

birth defect, 42
birthmark, 42
blind, 58
Bodhisattvas Realm, 12, 52
breast cancer, 63
Breast cancer, 30
breathing, 72
bronchitis, 43
Buddhism, 24, 53

C

cancer, 25, 36, 42, 57
Carl Jung, 10
chakra, 34
Christianity, vii
common cold, 37
complementary and alternative medicine, vii, 21
coronary heart disease, 30
Cosmic Realm, 12
cutting down the karma, 42
Cutting down the karma, 39

D

dementia, 32
Dissociative identity disorder, 37
drug addiction, 29

E

Ebola, 37
eczema, 31
eightfold path, 53
El Cantare, 3, 4
electric shocks, 38
exercise, 24

F

faith, 69, 70
fatigue, 25
forgiving love, 52
fundamental love, 52
Fundamental love, 56

G

gamble dependency, 29
gender identity disorder, 43
genetic factor, 27
gratitude, 57, 58
greed, 28, 65
guardian spirit, 13
guiding spirit, 13

H

Happy Science, viii, 1
Happy Science Medicine, 22
hatred, 29
Hell, 11
heredity, 27, 36
Hermes, 21

I

ignorance, 61
Ignorance, 30
ikiryo, 36
influenza, 37
Islam, 56

J

Jesus, 3, 7, 66, 69

K

karma, 22, 39, 73
karma reading, 42, 56
karmic law, 39

L

Law of Same Wavelengths' Attraction, 33
Law of the compensation, 39
leukemia, 22
light body, 14
Light Realm, 11, 52
Love, 2
Love Balance Sheet, 58
love incarnate, 52
love that gives, 52

M

metabolic syndrome, 29
Method of making a list of current worries, 61
mind, 17, 22
Moses, 4
Muhammad, 4
Multiple personality disorder, 37

N

Notion of Uncleanness, 66
nutrition, 25

O

optimalism, 63
optimism, 68
organ transplant, 15, 38

P

panic disorder, 43
Past Life Therapy, 7, 73
perfectionism, 62
perfectionist, 29, 64

pervasive development disorder, 40
phobia, 43
physical factors, 24
physical reading, 16
placebo effect, 69
possession, 23, 61
prayer, 70
presbyopia, 31
Principles of Happiness, 2
Progress, 2

R

Realm of Good, 52
Realm of the Good, 11
reincarnation, 6
rheumatic arthritis, 36
rheumatic disorders, 36
rheumatism, 34
Right Action, 60
Right Concentration, 68
Right Effort, 65
Right Livelihood, 60
Right Mindfulness, 68
Right Speech, 56
Right Thought, 65
Right View, 56
Rules of Attraction, 31
Ryuho Okawa, 1, 3

S

schizophrenia, 37
self-abasement, 29
Self-reflection, 2
sexual dependency, 29
sexual desire, 66
shopaholicism, 29
sleeping, 26
smiling, 57
soulmate, 40
spiritual body, 14, 15
spiritual views of life, 7, 31, 57
spiritually nurturing love, 52
Spiritually nurturing love, 60
stages of love, 52
stress, 22
stroke, 29
subconscious, 27, 31
suicide, 38

T

Tathagata Realm, 12, 53
the unconscious, 10
tumor, 25

U

universal unconscious, 69
Universal Unconscious, 10
ureteral stone, 31
Uterine cancer, 30
Uterine myoma, 30

W

wart, 25
willpower, 68
Wisdom, 2
workaholic, 29